A Penguin Special

TOBACCO:

THE TRUTH BEHIND THE SMOK

James Wilkinson graduated from King's College, London, with a degree in botany. After a year at Churchill College, Cambridge, he became science correspondent for the *Daily Express*. In 1974 he became science and air correspondent for BBC Radio News and in 1983 he became science correspondent for BBC TV News. He published *The Conquest of Cancer* in 1973. James Wilkinson is married with two sons and lives in Barnes.

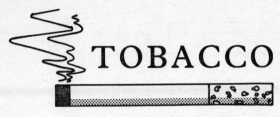

TOBACCO

The Truth behind the Smokescreen

JAMES WILKINSON

Penguin Books

Penguin Books Ltd, Harmondsworth, Middlesex, England
Viking Penguin Inc., 40 West 23rd Street, New York, New York 10010, U.S.A.
Penguin Books Australia Ltd, Ringwood, Victoria, Australia
Penguin Books Canada Limited, 2801 John Street, Markham, Ontario, Canada L3R 1B4
Penguin Books (N.Z.) Ltd, 182–190 Wairau Road, Auckland 10, New Zealand

First published 1986

Made and printed in Great Britain by
Richard Clay (The Chaucer Press) Ltd,
Bungay, Suffolk
Filmset in Monophoto Plantin by
Northumberland Press Ltd, Gateshead,
Tyne and Wear

For my sons Christopher and Matthew,

in the fervent hope that they are never seduced into the smoking habit by the tobacco industry

Contents

Acknowledgement

I would like to acknowledge the help given to me by the organization Action on Smoking and Health and its director, Mr David Simpson, who kindly read the manuscript and made many helpful suggestions.

1 *The World-Wide Epidemic*

The fact that smoking causes lung cancer and is a contributory cause of many other diseases has been recognized for over thirty years, yet cigarette manufacturers continue to promote their product, tobacconists continue to sell cigarettes, and the habit still kills many thousands each year in Britain and millions more around the world.

It is estimated that nearly six million new cases of cancer occur in the world each year. Of these about 15 per cent, or some 900,000 cases, are caused by tobacco. Lung cancer is the most frequently found cancer in men – well over 120,000 new cases a year.

Although the West is beginning to take small steps towards bringing the smoking epidemic under control, it is a very different story in many of the developing countries, where tobacco is a profitable crop and where sophisticated agreements between the tobacco manufacturers and governments, which go some way to limiting the industry's influence in the developed world, are not yet felt necessary. Two-thirds of new cases of lung cancer occur in developing countries, where smoking is very prevalent.

In Britain it is estimated that 100,000 people die prematurely each year from smoking. Some doctors have compared this death rate with the far smaller death rate for heroin addiction. Heroin addiction tends to kill more quickly and no one is belittling the evils of that drug, but the fact that smoking can take thirty or forty years to kill does not mean that it should be more acceptable in a civilized society.

In a speech at the Conservative Party Conference in October 1984, the junior health minister, Kenneth Clarke, said, 'dealing in addictive drugs is not a crime of passion or hot blood but a cold-blooded, premeditated act by people who know the drugs can kill'. He was talking of heroin. The same description can apply equally to those who make and sell cigarettes.

The American government's most senior drug official, Dr William

Pollin, director of the National Institute on Drug Abuse, has said he wants controls on tobacco promotion tightened up because it is a powerfully addictive drug. He believes tobacco could be eight times deadlier than excessive alcohol use and is more resistant to treatment than heroin addiction, which, he says, is also less likely to be fatal. He said, 'our society should seek some appropriate way to inhibit the present degree of freedom to push its most prevalent drug of abuse – nicotine'.[1]

Before we look in detail at the illnesses cigarettes cause and what is being done about the cigarette menace, let us first look at some figures. In Britain, at least, there is some cause for hope. People are at last beginning to recognize and act on the facts – and as a result

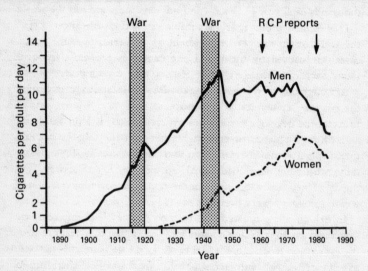

Figure 1

smoking is declining. In 1982, for example, smokers were for the first time in a minority in every socio-economic group, including male unskilled manual workers.[2] Among this group 57 per cent smoked in 1980. This had dropped to 49 per cent in 1982. Compared with ten years ago, the decline in smoking has been impressive. In 1972 52 per cent of men over sixteen smoked cigarettes. By 1980 42 per cent smoked cigarettes, by 1982 only 38 per cent of men smoked, and this fell further to 36 per cent in 1984. This means that smoking among men fell by over a quarter in this period.

For women the picture was slightly different. In 1972 41 per cent of women over sixteen smoked. In 1980 37 per cent smoked and by 1982 33 per cent smoked. There had again been a fall – but a smaller one. Smoking among women continues to fall very slightly.

Again, between 1980 and 1982 not only was there a decline in the number of men who smoked, but those who did smoke smoked fewer cigarettes. In 1982 the average weekly consumption of cigarettes among men had fallen to what it had been ten years earlier in 1972. The picture with women was not so encouraging. Those women who did smoke were smoking some 12 per cent more cigarettes in 1982 compared with 1972.

In 1984 men smokers over sixteen smoked an average of 115 cigarettes a week, compared with 120 in 1972.[3] Cigarette consumption per smoker had reached its peak in 1976 when men smokers smoked, on average, 129 cigarettes a week. During that same ten-year period cigarette smoking per woman smoker increased to 102 cigarettes a week in 1980 before beginning to decrease.

In terms of the number of cigarettes per smoker, Britain still has a long way to go to catch the world's greatest smokers – the Americans. Americans smoke 2,680 cigarettes a year per smoker. Japan is a close second with 2,600 cigarettes a year per smoker, West Germans get through 1,870 cigarettes a year, and British smokers 1,820.[4] Though smoking has declined generally in America, heavy smoking has increased. The proportion of American smokers who smoke more than twenty-five cigarettes a day has risen from 25 to 34 per cent among men and from 14 to 24 per cent among women.

There are one or two lone voices in government departments in Britain proclaiming the dangers of cigarettes, but they tend to go largely unheard in the corridors of power. The sale of cigarettes is so important a means of raising revenue that any substantial fall in sales could have a marked effect on revenue. Over the years the government's chief medical officers have been just about the only branch of the government machine which has repeatedly drawn attention to the havoc being caused by smoking.

There has been some action, albeit mild. In 1971 a voluntary agreement between the Department of Health and the tobacco manufacturers was reached. The manufacturers agreed to print on the side of cigarette packets WARNING BY HM GOVERNMENT: SMOKING CAN DAMAGE YOUR HEALTH, and to include on all advertisements for cigarettes the words 'Every packet carries a Government Health Warning'. This agreement has been renegotiated several times since then and extended to cover advertising and promotion of cigarettes.

In his annual report for 1983, Donald Acheson, the Department of Health's chief medical officer, said that cigarette smoking was the largest avoidable hazard in Britain today, causing about 100,000 deaths a year. He pointed out that ten years earlier, in 1972, one of his predecessors had described the cigarette as 'the most lethal instrument devised by man for peaceful use'. The new voluntary agreement reached that year between the government and the tobacco companies, he said, would lead to a reduction in the amount of tar each cigarette would contain and he welcomed this. But he added that, although this would help to reduce the incidence of lung cancer, it would be much less likely to affect the incidence of other tobacco-related diseases like coronary heart disease and diseases of the arteries.

One of the biggest falls in the number of smokers occurred just after the publication in 1962 of the first report by the Royal College of Physicians in Britain, which detailed the risks of smoking in a way which had not been done before. This resulted in a drop of 5 per cent in cigarette sales. However, because of the addictive nature of cigarettes, the slump in sales was followed by a slow drift back, until eventually more cigarettes than ever were being sold. A similar though smaller fall occurred after the Royal College of Physicians published a second report, nine years later.

Despite the publicity which followed the 1962 report, people still had a lot of misconceptions about the dangers of smoking. For example in 1967, a survey showed that three-quarters of all smokers believed that road accidents killed more people than smoking.[5] In fact smoking kills more than ten times that number. In 1967 over 80 per cent of smokers believed that smog and fumes were more important causes of lung cancer than smoking. Surveys in 1967 also showed up a belief among smokers which even now forms the basis of one of the arguments put forward by the tobacco companies whenever they are challenged about the dangers of smoking: 86 per cent of smokers believed that experts differed about whether smoking caused lung cancer. Thirty years later the tobacco companies are still referring to the 'controversy' over whether smoking causes lung cancer or not!

By 1971 it had become clear that there was enormous resistance among smokers to appreciating just what risks they were running, so the second RCP report set out the dangers in a particularly graphic way. The report portrayed the risk run by an individual smoker by comparing it with a lottery. Assume that smokers and non-smokers are drawing tickets from boxes in which there are two sorts of tickets. Some are left blank, others have the word 'death' written on them, meaning that the person who draws that ticket will die within the next ten years. Non-smokers aged thirty-five would draw from a box containing seventy-five tickets, one of which would be marked 'death'. A heavy smoker, on the other hand, would draw from a box containing one 'death' ticket for every twenty-two blanks.

Astonishingly, the 1971 RCP report revealed some remarkable ignorance about smoking even among medical students. Only half the smokers among them believed that smoking caused lung cancer; others rejected the claim on the grounds that the evidence was 'only statistical'. When the 1983 RCP report was published the experts had refined the message a little further. Now they were telling smokers that one in four of them would be killed by smoking, and that on average a smoker of twenty cigarettes a day would lose an average of five or six years of life.

A survey conducted as recently as February 1985 showed that though nearly all smokers now recognize the danger of smoking, fewer than half said they were worried about the ill effects of smoking on their *own* health. They had a belief that 'it won't happen to me'. Yet the facts are stark. Of 1,000 young adults who smoke regularly, one will be murdered, six will be killed on the roads, and 250 will be killed by tobacco.

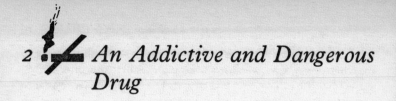

2 An Addictive and Dangerous Drug

If one had to single out one country to blame for the smoking epidemic in the West then perhaps it should be Spain. It was Spanish explorers of America in the early sixteenth century who introduced smoking to Western civilization, and much later it was the Spanish who invented cigarettes as a convenient way to smoke tobacco. English explorers in the sixteenth century also discovered smoking in the New World and brought the habit to England. It caught on in a big way – so big in fact that it was immediately seized on by Queen Elizabeth I as an easy way of raising revenue. And so the first tobacco tax was introduced – just 2*d*. a pound.

Even in those early days there was controversy about whether or not it was good for you. The French ambassador to Lisbon decided that smoking had beneficial medicinal properties and recommended it. His name was Jean Nicot – hence the word nicotine. Others were appalled by the habit. King James I was the first of the anti-smoking lobbyists. In his famous 'Counterblaste to Tobacco' (1604) he called tobacco 'hateful to the nose, harmful to the brain and dangerous to the lungs'.

Tobacco grew in popularity during the seventeenth century. It was smoked in pipes, chewed, and sniffed as snuff. Cigars were introduced into England at the beginning of the nineteenth century. Smoking got a further boost in popularity as milder tobaccos became available from Virginia, and the invention of the briar pipe made smoking tobacco easier and more pleasurable to some. Considering the lengthy history of smoking, cigarettes are a relatively recent phenomenon. They were introduced into England by soldiers returning from the Crimea and only really gained in popularity since the beginning of this century.

It was machine-made cigarettes which really helped the smoking epidemic take off. Cigarette-making machines were first used by an American, James 'Buck' Duke. His competitors had rejected the machines because they felt their customers preferred hand-rolled cigarettes. Buck Duke's machine was able to make 120,000 cigarettes a day, and because he was able to sell them more cheaply than his competitors, the smoking habit spread like wildfire. He bought out his rivals and formed the American Tobacco Company. In Britain cigarette manufacturers got together to resist his expansionist ambitions and formed the Imperial Tobacco Company, which included famous names like Wills of Bristol, John Player of Nottingham and Lambert and Butler of London. Finally, the two giants saw greater profit in co-operation than in competition and formed the British American Tobacco Company. Buck Duke was its first chairman.

However, the company was too big and a threat to free trade, so the courts decided it should split up again. Buck Duke's empire was not the only manufacturer. Philip Morris for example, now the maker of the world's most popular cigarette, Marlboro, began life as a London-based company making hand-rolled Turkish cigarettes in the nineteenth century. There are now six main companies, with interests in practically every country in the non-communist world: in addition to British American Tobacco, Imperial Tobacco and Philip Morris, there are R. J. Reynolds Industries Incorporated, American Brands Incorporated and the Rembrandt Group in South Africa, the parent company of Rothmans.

Cigarette smoking is so popular world-wide that the infrastructure to satisfy the craving is woven into the very fabric of society in such a way that if smoking were to stop tomorrow, the economies of scores of countries would collapse. In America smoking produces $14 billion a year in tax revenue. Two million people depend either partially or totally on tobacco for their livelihoods. In the southern states like Kentucky, Virginia, Tennessee, Georgia, Florida and Alabama there are some 600,000 farm families growing tobacco. Americans smoke a staggering 635 billion cigarettes a year. The American government recognizes the tobacco industry for the gold mine it is, and by a system of grants and subsidies guarantees a tobacco farmer a greater return on his crop than on almost any other crop. In 1979 the net profit from tobacco in North Carolina was $1,198 per acre, compared with $233 per acre for peanuts and $72 for soya beans. It is a similar story in the Third World, where the emphasis on tobacco is doubly shocking because so much land which could be growing food for the starving is dedicated to growing tobacco for home and export markets.

Hand in hand with the rise in cigarette smoking has come the rise in deaths from lung cancer. In Britain in 1920 there were 250 recorded deaths from lung cancer. By 1960 this had risen to 10,000. In America in 1930 3,000 people died from lung cancer. By 1962 the death toll had risen to 41,000.

People smoke because they have become addicted to nicotine. But there is more to it than that. There have been many studies to find out whether certain types of people are more prone to the addiction than others. It is not simply a craving for the drug itself which needs to be satisfied. Smokers tell how they become 'addicted' to the whole choreography of the smoking procedure, from taking the packet out of the pocket, lighting the cigarette, to the final stubbing out. It gives them something to do with their hands; it is ritualized fidgeting, which somehow becomes less noticeable and more acceptable because it is regular, routine and predictable.

Whether a person becomes a smoker or not is usually decided by the age of twenty. If someone is not a smoker at this age then he or she is unlikely to take it up. Psychologists have put forward a variety of ideas to suggest why people smoke. Some say it compensates for being weaned from the breast too early. Certainly one study has found that smokers who were able to give up smoking easily were not weaned until they were, on average, eight months old. Those unable to stop were weaned much earlier – at just over four and a half months.[6] It seems a neat idea – but other studies have not confirmed it.

There is also evidence of personality differences between smokers and non-smokers. Smokers tend to be impulsive, arousal-seeking, danger-loving, risk-taking people who do not like authority. They are also more prone to divorce, they have more car accidents, change jobs more often and tend to be more extroverted. Non-smokers, on the other hand, are said to be steadier, more dependable, quieter and less neurotic.

Similarly, there have been claims that some people are inherently predisposed to take up smoking, though smokers tempted to use this as an excuse for not being able to give up should not confuse it with lack of will-power! Studies of twins who have been brought up apart show that they are more likely to share the smoking habit if they are identical than if they are dissimilar.

In 1962 the Royal College of Physicians report *Smoking and Health* offered another reason why people smoke – it eases tensions between people. 'The proffering of a cigarette or tobacco pouch constitutes a gesture of friendship between negotiators or between assessors and applicants for a job.' The sentence already has a quaint and dated air about it. People proffering a cigarette in many social gatherings now would be looked at with mild horror.

Smoking increased significantly during the two world wars, (see Figure 1 on p. 12), showing that people turn to it at times of stress. There have been some strange claims about what would happen if it should become obsolete. Dr Johnson predicted that if this were to happen there would be an increase in madness. In the 1962 report the Royal College of Physicians felt it necessary to say 'there is no evidence to suggest that widespread discontinuance or diminution in the habit of smoking would result in any increase in neurotic disorders or physical disease'.

Whatever the psychological reasons which make people take up the habit and stay with it, there are also physical reasons to do with the properties of the active ingredient in cigarette smoke – nicotine.

Nicotine is certainly a potent drug. The amount of nicotine in one small cigar injected intravenously would be enough to kill an adult man. A smoker can absorb up to 10 per cent of this amount by smoking a cigar but the dose spread over about half an hour leaves sufficient time for at least some of the nicotine to be metabolized, lessening the impact of the poison. The smoke which a smoker draws through a cigarette contains between 0.4 to 3 mg of nicotine per cigarette, and up to 90 per cent of this may be absorbed by an inhaling smoker. From each puff of smoke a smoker may derive the equivalent of 0.1 mg of nicotine given intravenously.

Once in the body nicotine has effects which are many and complex. It acts on the nervous system and indirectly on the heart, the blood and blood vessels and the kidneys. The transmission of nervous impulses in the body from one cell to another is due to the release at the nerve endings of chemicals called neurotransmitters; these include acetylcholine and noradrenaline. Nicotine can mimic this action. Initially it stimulates the transmission of nerve impulses. Later it inhibits them. When a cat is injected with nicotine or is made to smoke, acetylcholine is released from its brain. The same thing happens when a cat wakes up. This release is accompanied by alterations in the electrical activity of the brain, indicating arousal. However, under some circumstances nicotine may also lower the activity of the animal's brain. In man, too, smoking can produce changes in the brain waves which indicate arousal, but it can also have a tranquillizing effect on the nervous system – for example, it depresses the knee-jerk reflex.

Nicotine releases the hormones adrenaline and noradrenaline from the adrenal glands and these affect the heart and blood vessels. Nicotine increases the heart rate and blood pressure and constricts the blood vessels. It also causes an increase in outflow from the heart. In smokers, after several hours abstinence, the heart rate can go up by 20 per cent or more. This can happen after the first cigarette of the day. However, in smokers with coronary heart disease the heart's output of blood may not rise; indeed, it may fall and the heart may beat abnormally.

Nicotine increases the concentration of fatty acids in the blood and also the stickiness of blood platelets. This can lead to clotting of the blood and may be involved in the formation of atheroma – the furring up of the walls of the blood vessels. Nicotine also helps stimulate the secretion of an antidiuretic hormone from the pituitary gland, which causes a temporary reduction in the production of urine.

Although nicotine is an addictive drug, smokers can have their daily nicotine intake reduced somewhat without their realizing it. If the nicotine content of cigarettes is lowered by 50 per cent then smokers increase their cigarette consumption by 10 per cent, which only makes up for some of the deficit. As with many drugs of addiction, the body adjusts to the nicotine intake and tolerance builds up, so the smoker has to increase his intake of cigarettes to achieve the same end result. People who inhale cigarette smoke for the first time suffer symptoms including palpitations, dizziness, sweating, nausea and vomiting. In man, tolerance takes some two or three years to build up, but rats injected with nicotine build up their tolerance very quickly and it persists for ninety days after the last injection.

As many smokers who have tried to give up know, cutting down or stopping smoking can lead to withdrawal symptoms, which include an intense craving for a cigarette, irritability, restlessness, depression and difficulty in concentrating. Apart from these psychological symptoms there are other physical effects which can be measured. Pulse rate and blood pressure fall, there can be gastrointestinal changes causing constipation, sleep can be disturbed and the ability to do certain tasks can be impaired. There are also measurable changes in the electrical activity of the brain.

Nicotine is just one of many thousands of substances in tobacco smoke. Tobacco leaves vary widely in their chemical make-up, depending on the species, where they are grown, which part of the leaf is used and how the leaves are dried, or 'cured'. There are three main ways of curing tobacco. Virginia tobacco is flue cured: the leaves are placed in barns and heated by furnaces for five to seven days. This preserves the sugar content of the leaves. Nearly all cigarettes sold in Britain are made from leaves cured in this way. Oriental tobaccos are cured in the sun, which leads to some loss of sugar, while Burley, Maryland and cigar tobaccos are air cured without heat for several weeks and as a result lose their sugars.

Each puff of a cigarette produces a mouthful of about 50 ml of dense smoke containing 50 mg of material, 18 mg of which is solid particulate matter, the rest being gases and vapours. The particulate matter is an aerosol of tar. Each droplet of tar is smaller than one ten-thousandth of a pin head. A smoker takes into his mouth a million million tiny droplets like this with each cigarette he smokes. After the smoker has exhaled, some 70 per cent of the tar is left behind in the airways and lungs. The nicotine which is dissolved in the tarry droplets enters the blood stream and is carried all over the body and especially to the brain. As a cigarette is smoked, many of the substances deposited on the tobacco as the smoke is drawn through get redistilled, and so the shorter the stub the stronger the smoke.

Tobacco smoke is intensely irritant. Some ten or more substances have been identified in smoke which are responsible for this effect, the most important of which is acrolein. They help cause the immediate coughing and narrowing of the bronchial tubes which occur after cigarette smoke is inhaled. They also slow up and stop the beating of the tiny hairs or cilia lining the airways in the lungs – the lungs' self-cleaning mechanism – and they also stimulate the bronchial glands to secrete increased amounts of mucus.

Many of the substances present in tobacco smoke have been isolated and painted on to the skin of mice to find out which ones cause cancer. The main culprits are thought to be the polycyclic aromatic hydrocarbons. Other substances help promote cancer by enhancing the action of chemicals which initiate it. These substances include phenols, fatty-acid esters and free fatty acids. Many of these are also irritants. The N-nitrosamine compounds are also thought to trigger cancer. One of them, N-nitrosonornicotine, has been identified in both tobacco smoke and unburnt tobacco, where it is present in concentrations of between 2,000 and 9,000 parts per billion – much higher than the concentration of other nitroso compounds found in meat and fish, where concentrations of only one part per billion are thought to present a potential health hazard. The presence of these substances in unburnt tobacco is thought to be one reason why chewing tobacco can produce mouth cancer.

Cigars and pipes are said to be safer than cigarettes, not because the smoke itself is less carcinogenic – in fact the opposite is true – but because it is not usually inhaled – the nicotine gets into the bloodstream by being absorbed through the lining of the mouth.

One of the gases present in tobacco smoke, carbon monoxide, is thought to be a particular health hazard because, although it has nothing to do with causing cancer, it starves the body of oxygen; in patients with angina or other heart or lung diseases this can be life-threatening. There are about 400 parts per million of carbon monoxide in cigarette smoke – a relatively high concentration. Because it has a much stronger affinity for haemoglobin than oxygen it is preferentially absorbed into the bloodstream; up to 10 or 15 per cent of a smoker's blood can be carrying carbon monoxide round the body instead of oxygen. Experimental animals exposed to carbon monoxide have been shown to have more atheroma in their blood vessels, and the same may well happen in man. It could also help to explain why smoking seems to interfere with the development of the unborn child.

In September 1985 a passenger who bought cigarettes at the duty-free shop at Gatwick airport found they had been tampered with. A note had been placed inside signed by the Animal Liberation Front, saying the cigarettes had been impregnated with cyanide. The tobacco company involved said later they thought it was a hoax, but there had been a series of protests in England organized by a militant lobby against the use of animals in research, and the traveller was, not surprisingly, horrified. Perhaps she would have been just as horrified had she realized that all cigarette smoke contains hydrogen cyanide. Cyanates derived from this hydrogen cyanide may impair heart function in smokers.

Cigarettes even contain radioactive chemicals like polonium 210. A report in the *National Academy of Sciences Proceedings* looked at the question of radioactivity in cigarette smoke and claimed that the smoke collects radioactive particles from the air and deposits them in the lungs. One expert, Dr Edward Martell from the National Centre for Atmospheric Research, claims that most lung cancer is caused by this radiation. He claims that smoking twenty cigarettes a day for forty years can result in a cumulative radiation dose of 38 to 97 rads of alpha radiation. Forty cigarettes a day could result in a dose of between 61 and 134 rads. He says there is a high probability that cancer can develop from exposure to between 80 and 100 rads. He also believes that radioactivity may well help cause cancer of the larynx, pharynx and oesophagus in smokers.

The first suggestion that smoking might lead to lung cancer has been traced back to 1898. Then, in 1914, a Dr Brinkman noticed that of 108 cases of lung cancer observed at the Leipzig Pathological Institute between 1900 and 1912, an unexpectedly large proportion were cigar makers and sellers, waiters and innkeepers – all occupations where you might expect there to be an excess of smokers. Thirteen years later, in 1927, a doctor addressing the Pathological Society drew attention to the increase in the number of lung cancers found at autopsy and suggested that cigarettes might be the cause. After ten more years, Professor Raymond Pearl, having studied the family history records of nearly 7,000 men at the School of Hygiene and Public Health of Johns Hopkins University, said, 'the smoking of tobacco was statistically associated with the impairment of life duration and the amount or degree of this impairment increased as the habitual amount of smoking increased'.[7] Others were not convinced, saying it was probably due to some other biological feature. Even ten years after he published his results, an editorial in the *American Medical Association Journal* said, 'extensive scientific studies have proved that smoking in moderation by those for whom tobacco is not especially contraindicated does not appreciably shorten life'. The journal had apparently been unconvinced by other papers which had been published on the subject, notably one study from Germany.

In 1947 the Medical Research Council in Britain called a meeting to consider possible reasons for the increase in deaths from lung cancer. It resolved to plan a large-scale statistical study of the past smoking habits of those with cancer of the lung, and to compare them with several control groups. So in January 1948 Dr Austin Bradford Hill and Dr Richard Doll began their study in twenty London hospitals. Dr Doll admits now that neither of them had much enthusiasm for the idea that tobacco might be a cause. Doll says he was more inclined to believe it might have something to do with the introduction of cars.

In 1949 they wrote their first paper on the subject, in which they reported preliminary findings on 649 male and sixty female cases. Their conclusion was: 'Smoking is a factor, and an important one, in the production of carcinoma of the lung.' They were advised against publishing the report until they had checked that their results could be reproduced outside London. Their paper was finally published in 1950, by which time similar results were being obtained with patients interviewed in Bristol, Cambridge, Leeds and Newcastle. By the end of the year eight studies had been published, all coming to similar conclusions, but they carried little weight with those who did not understand the science of epidemiology – studying the patterns of disease.

The following year, in November 1951, Sir Richard Doll began the famous study of British doctors which is still going on to this day. Doctors were chosen for the study because they were willing to co-operate and they were easy to trace. The results of this study showed that not only did smoking cause lung cancer but also that it contributed to heart disease. The first report of this study was published in June 1954. The figures were small. There were only 235 deaths from coronary thrombosis. But Bradford Hill and Doll concluded that 'the steady increase in mortality with the amount of tobacco smoking recorded suggests that there is a sub-group of these cases in which tobacco has a significant adjuvant effect'.

Two months after the paper by Bradford Hill and Doll was published, a similar study by Hammond and Horn was published in America. They studied nearly 5,000 deaths and concluded that cigarette smoking was a cause of both lung cancer and coronary artery thrombosis.

The secret was out at last. It had been difficult to extract because of the nature of the disease. Cancer can take thirty to forty years to develop in smokers. This can make it difficult to interpret results, as changes in smoking habits or types of cigarettes may not have a detectable impact on disease for many years. In China, for example, until recently lung cancer accounted for only 5 to 10 per cent of all cancer deaths, but smoking is now very widespread in China and experts are forecasting big increases in lung-cancer deaths there before the end of the century.

In America in 1915 cigarette sales averaged one cigarette per adult per day. By 1945 this had risen to 10 a day per adult. The results of this increase are only now becoming apparent, as lung-cancer rates in late middle-age and old age are still rising steeply, even though cigarette sales have remained roughly constant at about ten or twelve a day per adult since then.

The fact that the increase in disease lags behind the increase in smoking by thirty or forty years can lead to some puzzling anomalies. For example, in America tar levels have come down over the last twenty-five years but at the same time lung cancer rates have gone up. A recent report by the National Academy of Sciences and the National Research Council suggested that, in view of this, perhaps low-tar cigarettes were not effective. In fact the real reason for the anomaly is that the reductions in tar yields came too late to affect the long-term outlook for thousands of people who had already smoked high-tar cigarettes for many years before 1960.

Following the revelation in 1954 that lung cancer was definitely linked to smoking, the Home Affairs Committee of the British Cabinet discussed the issue. Minutes of one of its meetings made available under the thirty-year rule in 1984 revealed that the government decided to play down the link with tobacco partly because cigarette tax raised so much revenue. The tobacco industry also recognized the potentially serious effects this reported link between disease and smoking could have on its business and gave a grant of £250,000 to the Medical Research Council. This research grant also led the government to be cautious in any action it might take, because it feared losing the money were it to offend the cigarette companies! To his credit, the Marquis of Salisbury, a member of the government, did question whether it was exactly proper for the MRC to accept the grant from the tobacco industry.

An official government committee chaired by the government actuary, the Standing Advisory Committee on Cancer and Radio-therapy, also came to the conclusion that smoking caused lung cancer and suggested that young people should be warned. While the health minister accepted the suggestion, the Treasury financial secretary, John Boyd-Carpenter, did not. His entry in *Who's Who* does not suggest he has any scientific qualifications but he nevertheless questioned the evidence and suggested that the government's announcement of the report should emphasize that there might be other influences affecting the rates of lung cancer, not just smoking.

The result of all this was that on 12 February 1954 the health minister, Ian Macleod, played down the scientific conclusions in his statement to Parliament. He quoted the committee's findings and then said, 'I would draw attention to the fact that there is so far no firm evidence of the way in which smoking may cause lung cancer or of the extent to which it does so.' He also said more research was needed to determine further action. After the statement the Cabinet minutes record that Macleod briefed lobby correspondents, 'with the object of encouraging the press to maintain a due sense of proportion in their comments on his statement'.

The anti-smoking propaganda machine, starved of fuel and motivation by a nervous government anxious to protect its revenues, made only desultory efforts in the remainder of the 1950s. The Central Council of Health Education prepared pamphlets and provided lectures to talk on the subject but in the year 1958/9 they spent just £1,150 on these activities.

Advertising authorities too were cautious. A poster devised in 1958 showing a cigarette with smoke curling from it spelling the word 'cancer' was disallowed because the British Poster Advertising Association considered that the poster implied that one cigarette could cause cancer and this was misleading.

These low-key attempts in the 1950s to persuade people that smoking was bad for you achieved little. The event which really started the ball rolling occurred in 1962 – the publication of the first report on smoking and health by the Royal College of Physicians.

3 Smoking and Lung Cancer

The Royal College of Physicians set up a committee in 1959 to look at the smoking and lung-cancer issue because, although the link had been suspected for years, there were those who claimed, for example, that it was not smoking itself which caused lung cancer, but that both smoking and lung cancer might be the result of a third factor. Perhaps people who smoked were also more liable to develop lung cancer because of their genetic predisposition to the disease. There were also those who suspected that general air pollution might have a lot to do with lung cancer. The committee appointed by the College under its president Sir Robert (later Lord) Platt took three years to consider the evidence and publish its findings. When the report did finally appear its impact was sudden and dramatic. For the first time, unequivocal evidence was presented in a form everyone could understand, which showed that without a doubt cigarette smoking caused lung cancer.

The report pointed out that during adult life about 75 per cent of men smoked and 50 per cent of women. Men smoked on average nineteen cigarettes a day, women eleven. However, the report made it clear that the smoking habits of doctors were very different from the rest of the population. Heeding the results of earlier studies, doctors had been giving up in droves. In the ten years between 1951 and 1961 one in three doctors had given up the habit. A questionnaire to doctors revealed that in 1961 half of those questioned were non-smokers, compared with only a quarter of other men. Those who did smoke were also more likely to smoke a pipe. And, significantly, doctors developed far less lung cancer than the rest of the population. Britain was a good place to do this study because it had the highest rate of lung cancer in the world (as indeed it still has). The report concluded that cigarette smoking 'is the most likely cause of the recent world-wide increase in deaths from lung cancer'.

The report fleshed out its main conclusions with some chilling statistics about the real relative risks of dying of lung cancer depending on age and smoking habits. Heavy smokers – those who smoked twenty-five cigarettes a day or more – aged between thirty-five and forty-four had four times the death rate of comparable non-smokers. Heavy smokers aged seventy-five were twice as likely to die as non-smokers. It pointed out that the chances of a 35-year-old man dying before reaching the retiring age of sixty-five were 15 per cent for a non-smoker, but 33 per cent for a smoker. Looking at the death rate from lung cancer alone, it was calculated that someone smoking twenty-five cigarettes a day had a one in fourteen chance of dying of lung cancer between the ages of thirty-five and seventy-four. Furthermore, the report pointed out that smokers were also more likely to suffer from chronic bronchitis and heart disease (of which more later), and that smoking might be partly responsible for the persistent illness and deaths caused by tuberculosis.

The publication of the report had an immediate impact world wide. In America, especially, it was clear something had to be done, but President Kennedy felt himself to be in difficulties. He had only just beaten Richard Nixon in 1960 by a very narrow majority, largely through the help of the southern vote, which he had wooed by appointing Lyndon Johnson from Texas as his running mate. Hundreds of thousands of people in the South depended on tobacco for their livelihood, and taking strong action against smoking would only antagonize them. So he did what many governments do when they want to appear to be doing something about an issue even though they are simply buying time: he appointed his own committee of experts to look into the problem. The inquiry was carried out by the surgeon general, Dr Luther Terry. He very cleverly sought and obtained approval from the tobacco industry for the scientists appointed to serve on the inquiry. By so doing, if the inquiry found against smoking, the industry could not come back and say the experts were already biased. The inquiry studied some 6,000 articles and papers in some 1,200 journals and publications. The committee's conclusion, not surprisingly, was the same as that of the Royal College of Physicians: 'Cigarette smoking is a health hazard of sufficient importance in the United States to warrant appropriate remedial action.'

The surgeon general's report was published in 1964 and had an effect similar to that in Britain – sales of cigarettes fell. The year before publication 510 billion cigarettes had been sold. The year following publication sales had slumped to 495 billion, a relatively small drop perhaps, but one which had the cigarette manufacturers running for cover so that they could plan how to assault the market to restore their fortunes. They did not have to wait long. A year later sales had picked up again and reached 518 billion. Smokers' memories were short.

Since those early days of recognition, there have been three further reports from the Royal College of Physicians, each one coming to the same conclusions about the relationship between smoking and lung cancer, each one examining slightly different aspects of the problem, and each one trying to answer some of the objections which are raised from time to time by those with a vested interest in trying to weaken the public appreciation of the connection between smoking and lung cancer.

For example, some have said that the connection is not as strong as has been claimed, because scientists have had difficulty in inducing lung cancer in animals. There have been many experiments along these lines. One of the problems is that some animals have very efficient noses, which filter out the smoke before it reaches the lungs. Until the early seventies there was only one report of lung cancer having been initiated in mice made to smoke – and the disease took a different form to lung cancer in humans.

The 1971 Royal College report, *Smoking and Health Now*, cited one experiment in which twenty-four dogs, taught to inhale cigarette smoke directly into their lungs by tubes inserted in their windpipes so that the smoke by-passed their noses, had developed lung cancer similar to the human disease. This was after two and a half years of smoking seven unfiltered cigarettes a day. Dogs which had smoked filtered cigarettes in the same way for two and a half years did not develop lung cancer but displayed certain precancerous changes. Hamsters have also been used in experiments and when exposed to cigarette smoke some of these animals have also developed cancer of the larynx.

Those who sought to derive some comfort from the apparent difficulty scientists had found in reproducing human-type lung cancer in animals were warned not to be too confident. The 1971 report stated quite categorically, 'the direct evidence that cigarette smoking causes cancer of the lung in man is so clear that no experiments are needed to confirm it'. The report said that although animals were useful as a way of giving a pointer to the problems and might help in the testing of cigarettes modified to make them less dangerous, 'the ultimate measure of risk can be derived only from the prolonged study of the men and women who smoke them'.

The way cigarettes are smoked has a significant impact on the degree of risk the smoker runs. Inhaling increases the risk. The death rate from lung cancer in British doctors who said they inhaled was 80 per cent greater than in those who said they did not. The younger a smoker starts smoking apparently the greater the risk he runs. An American study has shown that men who had begun smoking before the age of fifteen ran five times the risk of dying from lung cancer compared with those who had begun smoking after the age of twenty-five. The more puffs a smoker takes of a cigarette, especially towards the butt end of the cigarette, the greater the risk of lung cancer. The risk increases if the cigarette is smoked quickly, and keeping the cigarette in the mouth also increases the risk.

There are three main types of lung cancer, two of which are common in cigarette-smoking patients. These are called squamous cell cancer, in which the cells resemble those of the skin, and 'small round-celled' or 'oat-celled' cancer. A third type known as 'adenocarcinoma' is less common in smokers.

Examining the lungs of smokers shows a variety of changes. In non-smokers with healthy lungs tiny little hairs called cilia line the windpipe. These hairs waft mucus continuously upwards towards the throat. In smokers these ciliated cells are often replaced by flattened cells without cilia. The deeper cells increase in number and many of them show changes which are pre-cancerous.

From the time a connection between lung cancer and smoking was first suspected there has always been a question mark over the connection in women. Superficially it seemed that women were less at risk than men. In Britain in the early 1970s deaths from lung cancer were five times as frequent in men as in women, whereas on average men smoked only about twice as much as women.[8] Studies had also shown that even when men and women smoked the same number of cigarettes, women had lower death rates from lung cancer.

The truth of the matter is that women smoke cigarettes differently from men. Older women in Britain started smoking later in their lives than men and they also inhaled less. In America women do not smoke cigarettes so far to the end as men. More women smoke filter-tipped cigarettes and lower-tar cigarettes. And at older ages, when lung cancer is most frequent, not so many women smoke as men.

In 1971 the Royal College of Physicians report concluded that 'if women continue to smoke more, to begin at an earlier age, and to smoke in the way men do, their death rate from this disease is likely to become nearly the same'. Figures since then have shown that the trend the doctors forecast then certainly seems to be occurring. Just as smoking during the previous twenty years increased more rapidly in women than in men, so lung cancer deaths increased too. In 1950 in America there were 4.6 deaths from lung cancer among women per 100,000. By 1982 the figure had risen to 20.9 per 100,000. In 1983, 17 per cent of all cancer deaths among women in America were due to lung cancer. In Washington state in 1980 lung cancer replaced breast cancer as the leading cause of death from cancer in women. A check on ten other states showed that in six of them lung-cancer deaths among women should shortly outnumber those from breast cancer, if they have not done so already. The same will be true in Britain.

Despite all the evidence, there are still one or two lone voices raised occasionally in the scientific community to question the validity of the claims that smoking causes lung cancer. The impact these voices have had on a smoking population anxious to justify the habit to themselves can be judged from a study carried out in the late 1960s which showed that nine out of ten smokers in Britain claimed that experts disagreed about the issue.[9] The facts show otherwise. By 1972 more than thirty investigations in ten countries had confirmed that smoking causes lung cancer. Just four of those studies covered a total of nearly one and a half million people investigated for four to ten years. The evidence proved that the risk of lung cancer increases with the number of cigarettes smoked.

Some people – and more particularly some tobacco companies – have sought to deny any connection by claiming that the evidence against smoking is 'only statistical'. The fact is that much of the evidence on the cause, prevention and treatment of all manner of human disease is 'only statistical' but this does not invalidate it. To suggest that there is no experimental evidence that smoking causes lung cancer is wrong. The biggest experiment of all demonstrates beyond doubt that millions of people who smoke often develop lung cancer while millions of others who do not smoke seldom develop the disease.

Another argument used by smokers, and in the past by some scientists, is that because of their genetic make-up people who smoke may also be more prone to develop lung cancer. However, there is direct evidence to refute this suggestion. British doctors who gave up smoking, for example, decreased their chances of getting lung cancer. Those who gave up did not have an inherently different genetic make-up compared with those who continued – rather they accepted the medical evidence. More persuasively, if people who smoked were also genetically more likely to develop lung cancer, why has the increase in the death rate been confined to the last fifty years – a time which coincides with the increase in cigarette smoking?

Then there is the argument that air pollution may be causing the increase. Indeed, in 1965 more than 80 per cent of smokers questioned considered that fog and fumes were more important causes of lung cancer than smoking. But while smoke in cities has been falling steadily, lung-cancer rates have been rising. Men are only slightly more exposed to air pollution than women, but the disease is much commoner in men. What of the suggestion that diesel-engine fumes are responsible? Again, lung cancer deaths began increasing before diesel-engine fuels were widely used, and anyway people who are more exposed to fumes from diesel engines do not show a significantly increased risk of lung cancer.

The recognition of the dangers of smoking, coupled with a variety of other influences including the introduction of filter cigarettes and, more recently, low-tar cigarettes, has had an impact. Death rates among middle-aged men in Britain levelled off and began to fall in the 1960s. A few years later something similar happened in older men. But in America, death rates have continued to rise in most age groups except in the very youngest, where there is a slight downward trend. In both countries lung-cancer deaths among women continue to rise.

The one encouraging trend is the decline in the rate of lung cancer in women in the younger age groups in Britain, although the numbers are small.

In 1971 the Royal College of Physicians report said that if people did not change their smoking habits, lung-cancer deaths among men would level out in the 1980s at some 35,000 to 40,000 a year, while the death rates from lung cancer in women would be about 10,000 to 15,000 a year, giving a total loss of life from lung cancer each year of between 45,000 and 55,000 deaths. A third of these deaths would be people below the age of sixty-five. In the event, people have been giving up – and the deaths from lung cancer are not quite as bad as the RCP predicted. Between 1981 and 1984 they averaged 29,693 for men and 10,403 for women: a total of about 40,000 a year. Taken year by year, total lung-cancer deaths among men of all ages dipped slightly in 1982 compared with the previous year, rose again in 1983 and fell by about 500 in 1984. Among women, however, there has been a steady rise.

Whether a person develops lung cancer or not may depend on other factors, not simply the number of cigarettes he or she smokes. For example diet seems to play a part. The body needs vitamin A to maintain the integrity of surface membranes. Too little vitamin A is associated with dry skin, night blindness and an undue susceptibility to cancer. Betacarotene, a precursor of vitamin A, is found in the diet in vegetables, chiefly carrots. Dietary inquiries have shown that where populations have a low intake of vitamin A there is a twofold increase in lung cancer. Doctors are now studying whether an increased intake of vitamin A in the diet can decrease the danger of getting lung cancer from smoking cigarettes.

Very thin people who smoke seem to be more prone to cancer of the lung than normal or fat people. And there are many substances which smokers may be exposed to at their work place which increase the chances of lung cancer developing. They include substances like asbestos, arsenic, chromates, nickel, chemicals like chlormethyl ethers, and radiation from uranium. Asbestos is a particularly nasty threat for smokers. One study showed that among 2,200 asbestos workers who did not smoke only two died from lung cancer. But among 9,590 smokers lung cancer caused 134 deaths. This means that an asbestos worker who smokes has his chances of dying from lung cancer

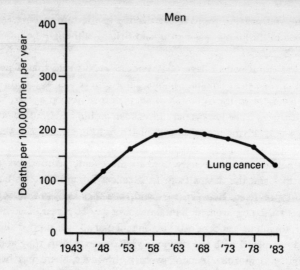

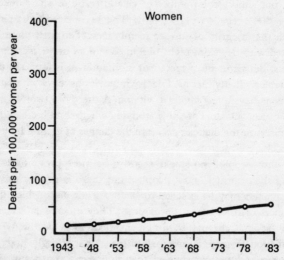

Figure 2

increased by ninety times compared with a non-smoker who doesn't work with asbestos.

Yet in the face of all the evidence, smokers have a remarkable ability to delude themselves. A survey carried out in 1983 by the Office of Population Censuses and Surveys revealed that most smokers, although realizing that smoking caused lung cancer, said they believed they would escape because they did not smoke enough. Half said they thought smoking could not be all that dangerous or the government would ban cigarette advertising.

Perhaps it is just because some people find smoking so difficult to give up that smokers try to reassure themselves by looking for any crumb of comfort they can extract from the various reports and surveys. The fact is that even after a lung-cancer operation nearly half the patients start smoking again if they survive.

Accepting that smoking is dangerous, what evidence is there of the benefit of giving up – especially if you have smoked for many years? The evidence is very encouraging. An American survey in 1984 looked at the risk of lung cancer among people who had given up smoking. It found that the risks of developing the disease among people who had given up for ten years were less than half those of people who had continued to smoke. The study involved over 7,000 lung-cancer patients from seven countries. Their smoking history was compared with 11,000 controls. The reduction in risk once a person had stopped smoking depended on how long he had smoked for. The risks after not smoking for ten years in both men and women who had previously smoked for less than twenty years were roughly the same as those for life-long non-smokers. And the doctors suggest that 'this should induce people starting to smoke regularly and short-term smokers to stop before changes become irreversible'. However, people who gave up smoking after forty years of cigarette use were still at substantially increased risk even ten years after giving up compared with those who had never smoked. In fact the report says they are unlikely ever to approach the level of risk found in those who have never smoked.

Lung cancer is not the only chest disease caused by smoking. Many smokers get what is known as chronic mucus hypersecretion. It is a response to the irritation caused by smoke and results in a persistent cough with phlegm – a form of bronchitis. It arises in the large airways and clears up when the smoker gives up. Post-mortem studies have shown that the lungs of smokers show enlargement of the glands in the bronchial tubes that produce mucus.

The other lung condition is far more serious and is known by the catch-all phrase 'chronic obstructive lung disease'. The tiny air passages become narrow and breathing becomes difficult. This is just as fatal as lung cancer and even more disabling. Doctors test for this by doing what is called a lung-function test. The patient is asked to blow into a tube as hard as he can. The machine records the maximum amount of air expelled during the first second after a deep breath. If it has fallen to about a litre the patient is usually disabled. The decline in lung function occurs over a period of decades and is irreversible. In some people lung function deteriorates particularly fast and in these people giving up smoking before the condition has gone too far is of crucial importance. If susceptible smokers could be identified early enough, they could be warned in time, but neither lung-function tests nor X-rays show up the condition until it is too late to do much about it. Doctors do not know how cigarettes cause this problem. It could have something to do with interference with the clearance of mucus from the airways, interference with the lungs' defences against infection, or interference with the balance of enzymes which maintain the lungs' integrity.

Each year about 30,000 men and women die from chronic obstructive lung disease – a combination of disorders which consist mainly of bronchitis and emphysema. Emphysema is a disease in which the minute air sacs in the lung break down giving rise to larger air spaces, so that the area of lung membrane available for oxygen to pass into the body and waste carbon dioxide to pass out is reduced.

Since the 1950s the number of deaths from chronic bronchitis among the general population has decreased steadily, probably because of improvements in the environment like clean air, improvements in general living conditions and also the advent of lower-tar cigarettes and filter-tipped cigarettes. But the situation is still bad. The effect of smoke on the lungs is easy to see even in the youngest smokers. Teenagers who smoke more than five cigarettes a day cough almost as much as adult smokers. The improvement which comes with filter cigarettes is shown by the fact that morning coughing has been found to be 6 per cent commoner in smokers of plain cigarettes than in smokers of filter-tipped ones.

The death rate from chronic obstructive lung disease is six times as great in smokers as in non-smokers, and those who smoke more than twenty-five cigarettes a day run twenty-five times the risk of non-smokers. Although giving up smoking will not necessarily enable structural changes in the lungs to be reversed, even at a late stage it will reduce the frequency of coughing and phlegm. For some reason, women do not seem to suffer from chronic obstructive lung disease to the same extent as men, even allowing for the differences in their smoking habits. In patients with moderately severe airflow obstruction stopping smoking will slow down the development of obstruction of the airways. The implication is clearly that the sooner smoking is stopped the better.

There are some people who have a genetic predisposition to develop emphysema. They lack a certain enzyme in their bodies which in normal people protects the lung. When absent, this enzyme, alpha antitrypsin, allows a second enzyme to digest lung tissue. People with this deficiency can start to suffer from emphysema as early as forty. Smoking has a serious effect on these people. Breathlessness can set in as young as thirty-two and the average age of death in these people if they smoke is forty-eight, as compared with sixty-seven in non-smokers with this condition.

There is one other lung condition which has been shown to be more common in smokers: collapsed lung or spontaneous pneumothorax. In this condition a small leak from the surface of the lung causes air to collect between it and the chest wall. This condition is more frequently seen in cigarette smokers. Both the strain of coughing and the presence of emphysema may contribute to this.

Lung disorders, and particularly lung cancer, may be the best-known diseases connected with smoking, but there is one disorder which claims even more lives than cancer among smokers: heart disease.

4 · Smoking and Heart Disease

More cigarette smokers die of heart disease than lung cancer. This does not lessen the importance of lung cancer as one of the main diseases directly caused by smoking; it is merely that in the country as a whole there are many more deaths from heart disease – indeed it is the biggest killer disease. The fact that relatively more cigarette smokers die of it shows that smoking is an important contributory cause.

What kills people is what is known as coronary artery disease. The coronary arteries carry blood to the heart muscle – the wall of the heart. Like other arteries elsewhere in the body, these can become narrowed by the deposition of fatty substances on the walls. This condition is called atheroma. When the heart muscle has to work hard it needs more oxygen. When the blood carrying this oxygen cannot pass through the narrowed vessels fast enough to deliver the oxygen, the patient gets a pain in the chest known as angina pectoris. It goes away when the patient is resting and the demands of the heart ease up. Sometimes when a blood clot forms and blocks one of these narrow arteries the heart may stop beating. Death may be immediate either because some of the heart muscle has died or because the heart's electrical activity has been interfered with. If only a small artery has been blocked then recovery may be complete.

Diseases of the heart and blood vessels account for a third of all excess deaths in smokers. Men under sixty-five years old who smoke twenty-five or more cigarettes a day are two and a half times more likely to develop coronary artery disease than non-smokers. The risk is not quite as high in older age groups, but this may well be because those who were particularly susceptible to heart disease have already died.

Some idea of the relative risk smokers face from heart disease can be judged by mortality figures taken from a study of British male doctors published in 1976. Among those doctors aged under forty-five who smoked twenty-five cigarettes a day there were 104 deaths per 100,000. Among non-smokers the number who died of a heart attack was just 7 per 100,000. Angina pectoris is also more common in cigarette smokers. Electrocardiograms taken during smoking may undergo changes, suggesting that there is a reduction in blood supply to the heart.

Smoking can also influence whether one survives after an initial heart attack. Heart attacks occur about two or three times more often in heavy smokers than in non-smokers, but smokers have four times the chance of dying suddenly following a heart attack. Among those who start smoking before the age of twenty and who smoke more than twenty cigarettes a day, the risk of dying from coronary heart disease is between three and five times the risk for non-smokers. One of the countries with the highest death rate for coronary heart disease in the world is Scotland. In Glasgow, for example, of the 290,000 people resident in the west of the city 60 per cent are regular smokers.

It is sometimes suggested that there are people with particular characteristics who are at special risk of coronary heart disease if they smoke, and there is some evidence for this. It seems that when cholesterol levels are low, for example, the effect of smoking seems relatively unimportant. In a study of British civil servants, the percentage of cigarette smokers dying of coronary heart disease was three times greater among those with high blood pressure and high cholesterol in their blood than among non-smokers with neither of these risk factors.[10] This is an important finding because it is easy to measure blood pressure and cholesterol; if patients in whom these levels are high can be identified, they can be made to see that advice about giving up smoking has a particular relevance for them.

As with lung cancer, there have been claims that the link between smoking and heart disease may not be causal but both may be linked to a third common factor. For example it has been suggested that the sort of person who smokes is also the same sort of person who develops a heart attack – the so-called type A personality: ambitious, extrovert, aggressive and competitive. But if heredity were responsible, the rates of heart attack would be unaffected by giving up smoking. In fact once someone has given up smoking, his risk of dying from a heart attack decreases steadily regardless of his personality type. The study of British doctors shows that between 1953 and 1965 there was a 6 per cent fall in deaths from all diseases of the heart and blood vessels among doctors, while among all men during this period there was a 9 per cent rise in such deaths.

Laboratory tests confirm that smoking has significant effects on the heart and blood. There is an increased tendency for the blood to clot after cigarette smoking. Smoking has long been known to precipitate bouts of rapid and often irregular beating of the heart which may cause palpitations, and indeed, laboratory tests have shown that nicotine increases the risk of disturbances in the rhythm of the heart. However, nicotine itself is unlikely to be the major cause of excess deaths from heart disease among cigarette smokers. A study of 145 cigarette smokers, forty-eight pipe smokers and twenty-seven non-smokers showed that both pipe and cigarette smokers had relatively high concentrations of nicotine in their blood compared with non-smokers, yet while cigarette smokers suffer a large excess of death from coronary artery disease, pipe smokers do not. It is possible, however, that because cigarette smokers get sudden high levels of nicotine in their bodies when they inhale, this might exert a toxic effect on the cardiovascular system.

Could the culprit, then, be carbon monoxide? Animal tests have shown that rabbits made to inhale air containing only 180 parts per million of carbon monoxide developed changes in their arteries similar to those found in men with coronary artery disease. The carbon monoxide seems to increase the permeability of blood vessels to cholesterol and this may encourage the formation of fatty deposits on the walls of blood vessels. Certainly, post-mortem studies of smokers have shown that the more cigarettes smoked, the greater is the deposition of fatty plaques.

Because carbon monoxide is carried round the body by red blood cells in preference to oxygen, in theory the heart muscle might well be starved of oxygen when a person smokes. There is evidence that this does happen – angina can occur during smoking, partly because the action of the nicotine makes the arteries constrict but also because the muscle does not get enough oxygen. There is also evidence that cigarette smokers tend to have more red blood cells, perhaps to compensate for those taken over by carbon monoxide. However, this itself may be harmful, as it tends to make the blood thicker and more prone to clotting.

So would there be any benefit to smokers in trying to reduce the amount of carbon monoxide in cigarette smoke? There could be, but a recent study published in the *New England Journal of Medicine* showed that men who smoke cigarettes with reduced amounts of nicotine and carbon monoxide do not have a lower risk of heart attack compared with those who smoke cigarettes containing larger amounts of these substances. However, the mere fact that carbon monoxide displaces oxygen in the blood shows that its presence in cigarette smoke inevitably poses a risk to people with pre-existing heart disease.

One study which tried to find out why smoking causes disease in the blood vessels looked at the way the body produced prostacyclin and the effect smoking had on its production.[11] Prostacyclin dilates the blood vessels and also inhibits the aggregation of platelets. Clearly, if smoking were found to result in a decrease in the amount of prostacyclin produced in the body, this could help explain two of the effects known to be associated with smoking: first, an increased tendency for the blood to become viscous and clot, and second, a tendency for the blood vessels to constrict after smoking. The amount of prostacyclin in the urine of twelve smokers was compared with that of twelve non-smokers. The results showed that in smokers there was a significant decrease in the prostacyclin present in the urine after they had smoked. The authors concluded that this reduction of prostacyclin after smoking 'may be a factor in the development of accelerated cardiovascular disease'.

Another suggestion concerns the role of lead in the blood. The British Regional Heart Study, which looked at the big differences in the death rate from heart disease in different parts of the country, discovered that the concentration of lead varied significantly from region to region. The highest concentrations were found in soft-water areas, which tend to have a relatively high level of heart disease. Cigarettes and alcohol contribute lead to the body, and the doctors who carried out this study concluded that 'for those individuals who drink and smoke heavily on a daily basis our evidence indicates that blood lead concentrations may typically increase over 50 per cent as a consequence'.

In 1971 the Royal College of Physicians report on smoking concluded that if people gave up smoking, the death rate from coronary artery disease could be reduced by 25 per cent in men aged between thirty-five and sixty-four and by 20 per cent in women – saving the lives of some 7,000 men and 1,500 women in this age group.

And it is never too late to give up, even after a heart attack. Indeed, research has shown that survivors of a heart attack who continue to smoke are twice as likely to die of a second heart attack than those who give up. In fact stopping smoking may be the most effective single means of ensuring protection against a heart attack. Patients who give up smoking after a heart attack can add, on average, up to six years to their lives.

The reasons why giving up smoking is so effective are not clear. It does not seem to make any difference to the atheroma which has already been laid down in the coronary arteries. A study of nearly 400 patients undergoing routine heart operations showed that there was no difference in the severity of coronary artery disease between current smokers and those who had given up smoking perhaps five or ten years previously. The coronary atheroma had not regressed. So the reduced incidence of repeat heart attacks in those who have given up shows that the beneficial effect must be due to the removal of some other factors. Doctors have suggested that these factors could include lower carboxyhaemoglobin concentrations, reduced blood viscosity, a reduction in the stickiness of platelets or perhaps a reduction in the risk that the heart may have its electrical activity interfered with.

The benefits of giving up last for many years and the reduced risk of dying from a heart attack is noticeable very soon after giving up. So strongly do some doctors feel about the stupidity of smoking after treatment for heart disease that one doctor at a London hospital has said that, apart from emergencies, he was refusing to carry out any more bypass operations on people who refused to give up smoking to improve their quality of life. He said that patients who continue to smoke after surgery made the doctors' efforts useless. He pointed out that there were plenty of patients on the waiting list who were willing to give up – and they should have preferential treatment.

Smoking is such a powerful addiction that it is perhaps somewhat unfair to lay too much blame on those who simply cannot give up despite the added incentive of having suffered a heart attack. A survey of sixty-six smokers who had had a heart attack showed that 38 per cent of them began smoking again while they were in hospital – often getting their cigarettes from visitors who brought them in with them – and most continued smoking when they left hospital. However, patients with the more severe heart attacks were the least likely to begin smoking again.[12]

Angina can also be an incentive to stop smoking, not only because patients are at risk of a heart attack but also because smoking can actually interfere with their drug treatment. A study by a London hospital has shown that drugs were found to be much more effective when the patients had given up smoking.[13] Stopping smoking increased the effect of the drug on heart rate, exercise tolerance, and the frequency of angina.

From all the evidence, then, it is clear that stopping smoking is the single most effective way of protecting oneself against heart disease – the biggest killer in the developed world.

Lung cancer, other chest diseases and heart disease may be the best-known illnesses caused by smoking but they are by no means the only ones. It is hardly surprising that when such a complex mixture of chemicals as is contained in cigarette smoke circulates in the blood-stream, the effects are widespread. There are links between smoking and cancer elsewhere in the body, and also between smoking and trouble in blood vessels far removed from the heart – trouble which can have devastating consequences for the smoker.

Consider first what is known as peripheral vascular disease. The sort of furring up of the arteries which occurs in the heart, and which leads to a blocking of the blood vessels and a heart attack, can also occur in the small blood vessels. This can restrict the blood flow to parts of the body, especially the legs, which can result in pain when walking and pain in the feet at rest. Eventually, gangrene may set in, making amputation necessary. Over 95 per cent of patients with arterial disease of the legs which causes pain when walking are reported to be smokers. A survey in one health service region in England showed that in 1981 225 people had amputations of lower limbs due to impaired circulation. In the same region only 32 people had their legs amputated because of injury.

Arterial disease caused by smoking can also lead to a narrowing of the carotid arteries supplying the brain, which can lead to strokes. Occasionally a damaged artery in any part of the body can blow up like a balloon to form an aneurysm, which may burst, causing a fatal haemorrhage. One study has shown that heavy smokers run a 70 per cent greater chance of dying of a stroke than non-smokers. Indeed, more than 90 per cent of patients suffering from any of these arterial diseases have smoked at least twenty cigarettes a day for twenty years or more. Very few have never smoked.

A variety of cancers has been associated with smoking, especially cancer of the mouth, pharynx, larynx and oesophagus. The more cigarettes smoked, the greater the risk, but it is not confined to cigarette smokers. Pipe and cigar smokers are equally at risk of these diseases. With cancer of the mouth and larynx, there is also an association with heavy drinking and it is clear that alcohol may be a contributory cause. Cigarette smokers run about twice the risk of bladder cancer compared with non-smokers. Cancer-causing substances have been found in the urine of smokers – metabolized products of the amino-acid tryptophan. These substances declined when smokers stopped smoking. There seems to be a link between smoking and cancer of the pancreas and also with cancer of the cervix. A recent review of the evidence in the *American Journal of Epidemiology* showed that of twelve studies examined, all but one found there was an association between smoking and cervical cancer. The link seems to hold good even when other factors are taken into consideration, such as age at first intercourse, the use of the pill, number of sexual partners and so on. The more a woman smoked, the greater was the risk.

The moment a teenager tries his first cigarette he knows the effect smoke can have on the stomach. It makes him feel distinctly sick. Adult smokers may not realize it, but smoking can have a continuing effect on the stomach and can cause ulcers. Heavy smokers are particularly at risk. A heavy smoker tends not to secrete so much pancreatic juice, which normally helps to neutralize the acid entering the duodenum from the stomach. Too little pancreatic secretion can lead to too much acid in the duodenum, resulting in the formation of an ulcer.

A survey in America has shown that peptic ulcer is twice as common in male smokers as in non-smokers and about one and a half times as common in women smokers.[14] Smoking can interfere with treatment. One study has shown that among patients who gave up smoking when advised to do so after starting treatment for their gastric ulcer, the size of the ulcer was reduced by 78 per cent. In those who continued to smoke, the ulcer was reduced in size by only 58 per cent. In some patients who continued to smoke, the ulcer actually grew in size. A study at the University of Dundee goes some way to explaining why this happens. In a group of smokers undergoing treatment for ulcers it was found that if they smoked, nocturnal acid secretion in their stomachs increased by 91 per cent and pepsin secretion by 60 per cent compared with patients who did not smoke while receiving treatment. Once an ulcer has healed, smoking increases the chances that it will recur. Indeed, it has even been suggested that one of the most effective treatments for duodenal ulcer may be to give up smoking. It may even be more effective than drug treatment.

The catalogue of diseases caused by smoking does not end there. Smokers are more likely to have inflammatory disease of the gums, possibly because they tend to be less careful about oral hygiene. Pipe smokers are just as prone to mouth disorders as are cigarette smokers. The presence of gum disorders like chronic gingivitis may also help explain another finding – that smokers are more likely to have had all their teeth extracted compared to non-smokers.

Smoking can also trigger migraine attacks. Oddly, women aged forty-five to sixty-five who suffer from migraine have a lower mortality than those who do not have migraine. This may well be because migraine sufferers recognize that smoking can trigger an attack and so avoid smoking. A survey at London's Charing Cross Hospital found that smokers had more frequent and more severe attacks of migraine. There was a tenfold drop in the number of attacks once patients had given up smoking.

Cigarette smokers are more likely to suffer from pulmonary tuberculosis than non-smokers and smoking may encourage the recrudescence of an old tuberculous infection.

Then there are the rare conditions which seem to be linked to smoking. Tobacco amblyopia is a rare cause of blindness which has been attributed to heavy smoking, particularly of pipes and cigars. There is a suggestion that damage to the optic nerve may be connected with the combined effect of the toxic action of cyanides absorbed from tobacco smoke and a vitamin B_{12} deficiency. And smoking may be an important factor in the cause of an uncommon skin condition called palmoplantar pustulosis, which is characterized by sterile yellow pustules that fade into brown patches (macules) lying in scaly areas. Smoking may also affect other more common inflammatory skin conditions like hand dermatitis and psoriasis.

For smokers unlucky enough to need an operation, smoking itself can increase the risk of surgical procedures. Nicotine increases the demand of the heart for oxygen by speeding it up and carbon monoxide decreases the supply of oxygen, so smoking places an extra burden on the heart during surgery. Stopping smoking for twelve to twenty-four hours before an operation can reduce the risk. However, this is not the only problem for smokers. They tend to have respiratory problems as a result of their addiction and smoking also reduces the immune system, making them more prone to post-operative infection, especially chest infections. Doctors prefer patients to give up smoking for six weeks before an operation.

If more proof were needed of the way smoking saps good health the figures for absence due to sickness provide it. One survey has shown that people who smoked more than twenty cigarettes a day lose twice as much time off work compared with non-smokers.[15] Smokers under forty-five make more demands on the medical services compared with non-smokers and they spend more time in hospital both as out-patients and in-patients. They also go to the doctors' surgery more often. Smokers generally tend to weigh less than non-smokers. Once a smoker stops smoking, he may put on weight. British doctors who stopped smoking gained an extra four pounds on average. They had to take more care with their diet than those who had never smoked, but ten years later they were, on average, only one pound heavier. The weight gain may be due to increased appetite after giving up smoking, although there is some suggestion that non-smokers tend to eat less than smokers. Stopping smoking can cause a number of changes in the metabolism and it could be this which accounts for the weight gain. Those smokers who try to use weight gain as an excuse for not giving up should not delude themselves into thinking this is a valid health reason for continuing smoking. The risks of smoking far outweigh the risks of being a little overweight.

Smoking is, or should be, of particular concern to women, not only because of the direct health effects on themselves but almost more importantly because of the risk they are exposing their babies and children to. If a woman wants to become pregnant she will find that if she smokes she is more likely to be infertile, or at least that she may take longer to conceive than women who do not smoke. Pregnant women who smoke have a small increased risk of spontaneous abortion, bleeding during pregnancy and of developing various placental abnormalities.

Women who smoke tend to become menopausal more quickly than

those who do not. One study has shown that women who have never smoked reach the menopause at an average age of 52.4 years.[16] Those who smoked between one and fourteen cigarettes a day reached the menopause at 51.9 years, and those who smoked thirty-five or more cigarettes a day became menopausal at 50.4 years. However, smoking has a real impact at an earlier age, not only on the woman herself but on any children she may want to bear

There have been several surveys on the smoking habits of women to try to find out why they smoke and why, among younger age groups, the incidence of smoking has continued to rise until now almost as many young women smoke as young men. Most surprising of all, nurses tend to smoke a lot. The Scottish Health Education Group found that women apparently hold short-term perspectives on their own health – they smoke to help them get over short-term pressures – but they hold long-term perspectives when considering the health of others. The women seemed happy to use cigarettes themselves to suppress their own irritability, in order to promote family harmony.

Anti-smoking campaigns have been aimed specifically at women. They have had a measurable but only temporary effect on smoking habits.

Women who smoke tend to favour the birth-control pill as a method of contraception – and it is they who bear the brunt of its side effects. The risk of heart attacks, strokes and other cardiovascular diseases is increased by approximately tenfold in women who both smoke and are on the pill compared with women not on the pill who do not smoke. This effect is more marked in women over forty-five and somewhat less in women under thirty-five. Doctors no longer prescribe the pill to women over thirty-five if they can help it, because the risk of the pill even among non-smokers increases after this age.

But almost more important than the risk to women themselves is the risk faced by the babies of smoking women both before and after birth. Babies born to women who smoke are on average up to half a pound lighter than those born to non-smokers. They are also more likely to be born premature. Mothers who smoke are, on average, two or three times more likely to have premature babies (those weighing less than five and a half pounds) compared with those who do not. The more cigarettes the woman smokes, the greater the chance of having a premature baby. These very light babies tend to catch up with normal-weight babies and when they are a year or so old there is little difference between them, so it seems that while they are in the womb something holds them back from developing normally.

The health of light-weight babies is at greater risk than that of normal-weight babies. They are more likely to die soon after birth. Mothers who smoke are more likely to have a miscarriage and to have a stillborn baby than non-smoking mothers. A study in Sheffield found that of over 2,000 pregnancies, nearly 8 per cent of mothers who smoked during pregnancy lost their babies, compared with only about 4 per cent of mothers who did not smoke.[17] Spontaneous abortion rates increase according to the number of cigarettes smoked.

There are two possible reasons why babies in the womb of smoking mothers are stunted. One contributory factor could be that carbon monoxide becomes more concentrated in the baby's blood than in the mother's, so effectively starving the baby of oxygen. However, placental blood-flow could also be reduced. Nicotine acts on the mother's brain, making it release the hormone oxytocin, which causes a contraction of the uterus. By compression this could reduce the flow of blood to the uterus and the placenta. Doctors have also found that in mothers who smoke more than twenty cigarettes a day, the baby's blood is 30 per cent more viscous.

There is incontrovertible evidence that it is smoking and nothing else which causes low birth-weight infants, because studies have shown that when mothers who smoked during their first pregnancy subsequently gave up and then had a second baby, the second baby weighed, on average, 169g more than the first. Similarly, when a mother took up smoking during her second pregnancy, having abstained during her first, the second baby weighed less than the first.

Animal studies have also shown that smoking can affect pregnancy. Pregnant rabbits exposed to carbon monoxide such that 16 to 18 per cent of their haemoglobin was in the form of carboxyhaemoglobin showed a much higher stillborn rate than normal, and they also gave birth to lighter offspring than normal.

Social class plays a part in the effects of smoking during pregnancy, though women smokers from all classes have lighter babies than normal. The risk of the baby dying only increased in the lower socio-economic groups – probably because better-off mothers had better nutrition and other advantages during their pregnancy. The risk of a baby dying at or soon after childbirth depends on the mother's smoking habits after the fourth month of pregnancy. If a woman has given up smoking by the fourth month then the outlook for her baby is as good as if she had never smoked. The effect of smoking on babies persists after birth. Smokers tend to stop breast feeding earlier than non-smokers and this may be because heavy smokers have less prolactin – a pituitary hormone which initiates lactation – in their blood than non-smokers.

There is also a suggestion that there is an increase in congenital malformation of the heart in children up to the age of seven who were born to mothers who smoked.

With this catalogue of potential disasters it is surprising that so many women still do smoke. In fact women seem to find it particularly difficult to give up. Even when initial efforts are successful, the relapse rate among women smokers is twice as great as in men. Women who stay at home while their husband is at work and their children are at school seem to find it particularly difficult to give up.

There is one other aspect of smoking and health which at first sight might not seem of importance – the risk that people can get burnt. Yet surprisingly, cigarettes and smoking materials are a major cause of fires which claim hundreds of lives a year. Smoking is believed to be the cause of about half the fires the fire brigade has to deal with. Between 1970 and 1980 in Britain there were 7,400 non-fatal casualties and 1,988 deaths in fires started by smoking materials. Every year the fire brigade in Britain attends 10,000 fires in occupied buildings which have started as a result of smoking. Between 1978 and 1980 the number of deaths caused by smoking materials or matches was up by about 60 per cent compared with a two-year period in the early seventies, even though cigarette sales had declined between 1972 and 1980. One reason could be the increasing use of flammable materials in upholstery.

In America it is a similar story. Cigarettes cause over 56,000 fires a year and 2,000 deaths. So concerned are the American authorities that Congress set up a three-man committee to investigate whether cigarettes should be made 'fire-safe', that is they would go out automatically if they are unsmoked (at the moment chemicals are added to make them burn by themselves). Not surprisingly, the tobacco industry is against the idea, but, aware of the danger of flammable materials, it recently contributed $73,000 to the technical development programme of the Upholstered Furniture Action Council, which is working to make furniture more flame-resistant.

It is not just homes which are at risk. In China an American oil consultant was sentenced to eighteen months in jail and fined for starting a fire accidentally in his hotel room. He fell asleep in bed and the lighted cigarette set his room on fire. Though he escaped, ten people died. A fire on board an Air Canada DC9 which killed twenty-three people was thought to have been started by a cigarette left in the lavatory. There were calls for a ban on smoking in aeroplanes but the more cautious pointed out that smoking was such a strong addiction that if it were banned some people would go to extraordinary lengths to conceal they were smoking, which could prove an even greater hazard. The fire tragedy few people will forget, thought to have been caused by a discarded cigarette, occurred in the Bradford football stand in 1985 when fifty-six people were killed. Surveying the wreckage, the chairman of Bradford City Football Club said, 'If people did not have the dirty, filthy habit of smoking there would be fifty-six people alive today.'

6 *So You Can't Give It Up?*

If smoking were not so addictive it would be easy to give up. Some manage to give up with relatively little difficulty. Others try time and again but eventually relapse because their willpower is not as strong as their craving. There have been all manner of methods devised to help people give up, from group clinics to hypnosis and alternative ways of getting nicotine into the bloodstream so that the desire for cigarettes is reduced. However, despite the interest from smokers in trying to give up there has been precious little official help from the medical authorities or the government to make it a national campaign.

In 1971 the Medical Research Council and the Social Science Research Council set up a committee to advise on research into ways to cut the number of smokers. A research project into the psychology of smoking and another into the smoking habits of school children were initiated and the results were published in 1975. A new project was set up in 1973 to study ways of preventing children from starting to smoke, but it never published a report.

Since then there have been innumerable surveys into how and why people smoke. However, the surveys themselves are of little benefit unless the results are acted upon and new schemes for encouraging people to give up smoking are devised. Doctors themselves often feel inadequate when faced with a patient who wants to give up smoking. In America a group of 490 doctors from Massachusetts were surveyed about their attitudes and beliefs about health education. Ninety-three per cent thought that eliminating cigarette smoking was very important for promoting health but only 58 per cent felt very prepared to counsel patients about how to give up, and only 3 per cent thought they were very successful in helping patients to give up. Yet smokers are crying out for help.

In Britain some 92 per cent of smokers now accept that there is a connection between smoking and ill health. Seventy per cent of smokers have made one or more attempts to give up smoking during the previous ten years. Some indication of how concerned smokers are is given by the sales of low-tar and filter cigarettes; 85 per cent of smokers now use tipped cigarettes and 90 per cent smoke cigarettes with a tar content of less than 20 mg. Yet help is slow in coming. The third Royal College of Physicians report on smoking, *Smoking or Health*, said,

The recommendation which we made five years ago that the DHSS should set up a joint committee with the MRC to advise on staff, techniques, record keeping and research in [smoking withdrawal] clinics has been ignored. For this reason we know no more now than we did then about the potential clientele for such clinics or about reasons for differences in success rates between different doctors. No adequate trials have been mounted to discover how low a nicotine intake smokers can gradually become adapted to without increasing their cigarette consumption, or whether those who do accept very low nicotine yields can subsequently stop smoking without difficulty. We repeat our recommendations that steps be taken to ensure that the efforts of existing clinics are not wasted by lack of objective study of their methods and results. If this were properly organized, a higher level of achievement might be attained which could justify establishing more such clinics.

The report also pointed out some of the results of surveys into giving up smoking. For example, the longer a person has stopped smoking the less likely they will be to start smoking again. Of those who have given up smoking for less than a year nearly 40 per cent will start again within two years. Of those who have given it up for between one and two years, only 19 per cent will start again. Of those who have abstained for more than two years only 5 per cent will relapse.

One product which does seem to have had an impact in helping people to give up is a chewing gum containing nicotine known as Nicorette, first introduced in Britain in 1980. It releases nicotine which is absorbed into the bloodstream through the lining of the mouth. Trials have shown that it does help wean smokers off cigarettes, but it seems to work better when it is used within the setting of an anti-smoking clinic. Researchers at the Addiction Research Unit at the Institute of Psychiatry in London have developed a nasal solution containing nicotine which delivers nicotine to the system faster than chewing gum. The researchers say this might be helpful to smokers trying to give up the habit.

However, despite the aids to giving up smoking it is clear that much more success could be achieved with a concerted and officially backed and funded programme. It is ironic that more than thirty years after the scientific recognition of the dangers of smoking one of the country's leading epidemiologists, Sir Richard Doll, should still feel it necessary to make a plea for controlled trials to be set up into the various different ways of giving up smoking.

If smokers cannot give up, there are several ways in which they can reduce the risk they run from smoking. Switching from cigarettes to a pipe is one. Pipe smokers tend not to inhale and so their lungs are not exposed to the tar in cigarettes which gives rise to cancer. Heavy cigarette smokers do sometimes continue to inhale after switching to a pipe, cancelling out any benefit such a change might produce for them. Switching to filter-tipped cigarettes or low-tar cigarettes is also a good idea, as the tar delivery is lower. The 1977 Royal College of Physicians report said that from the limited studies carried out, smokers can accept cigarettes with a wide range of nicotine levels. Most smokers find a cigarette containing as little as 1 mg nicotine quite satisfying. The report suggested that it was desirable, therefore, to sell cigarettes with nicotine yields of less than 1 mg, provided the nicotine level was associated with tar levels below 15 mg, and recommended that there should be regulations to this effect. It urged that regulations should also limit the amount of carbon monoxide produced by cigarettes to the lowest amount practicable.

Adding a filter to the end of a cigarette reduces the amount of the tar that gets into the lungs. In 1975 87 per cent of all cigarettes sold were filter-tipped. This, combined with the fact that tar yields in filter-tipped cigarettes have also been reduced, meant that the average smoker was exposed to 43 per cent less tar in 1975 than in 1965. In the early 1950s tar yields were very high. But they began to come down in the second half of the fifties and have been dropping ever since. In 1966–71 there was an average of 30.4 mg of tar per cigarette. This had halved by 1982. Nicotine and carbon monoxide levels have also come down. Nicotine has been reduced from 2.03 mg per cigarette in 1955–61 to 1.28 mg in 1974 – a cut of 37 per cent. Carbon monoxide fell from 20.6 mg in 1955–61 to 16 mg in 1976 – a fall of 22 per cent. By 1979 there had been slight rises in both the nicotine and carbon monoxide levels in cigarettes, mainly due to the increase in the sale of kingsize cigarettes.

It has been shown that without doubt altering smoking habits helps to cut down ill-health. An American study demonstrated that men who had changed to filter-tipped cigarettes during the previous ten years reduced their risk of getting lung cancer by 40 per cent compared with men who did not switch.

Making a cigarette with a low tar content can be achieved in different ways. The tar content depends on how the tobacco is cured, for example, and on how porous the paper is: the greater the amount of air drawn in through the sides of the cigarette during a puff the less smoke there will be in the mouthful of smoke taken in. The risk of smoking seems to be more dependent on the length of time a person has smoked for than on the amount he has smoked. For example, it has been established that smoking two packets a day for twenty years is less hazardous than smoking one packet a day for forty years.

By the early seventies it became clear that smokers needed some guidance on tar and nicotine levels, even though these had been coming down slowly anyway. Tar tables were published for the first time in 1973. By 1975 cigarettes were classified into groups according to tar delivery. By 1982 low-tar cigarettes accounted for nearly 20 per cent of the market.

In 1983 the third report by the Independent Scientific Committee on Smoking and Health recommended that over the four-year period 1984-7 the amount of tar produced by cigarettes should be reduced at the same rate as between 1979 and 1983. This would produce an average tar yield of approximately 13 mg per cigarette by the end of 1987 (the target at the time the report was published was 15 mg per cigarette by the end of 1983). The report also recommended that every new brand introduced on to the market should, in future, deliver less than 13 mg tar per cigarette and that no new brands should be introduced with carbon monoxide yields exceeding about 15 mg per cigarette. Before this there had been no ceiling. The government response to the report was given by the junior health minister, John Patten, who said the committee's recommendations would be borne in mind in the course of the government's discussion with the tobacco companies on a new voluntary agreement on product modification. If the minister were in any doubt about the strength of feeling in the medical profession about the need for some more positive action, this should have been dispelled by the 1983 Royal College of Physicians report, which concluded,

Whilst looking always for a government lead which will aim to encourage smokers to stop smoking altogether, a tar-reduction programme should certainly be part of government strategy. Further reductions in the tar and nicotine deliveries of cigarettes could be made, and enforced if necessary by legislation.

However, progress has been slow. In January 1985 two of the leading epidemiologists in this field, Doll and Peto, stressed once again the ease with which the government could reduce the tar content of tobacco. They pointed out that low tar levels did not hit growers, manufacturers, distributors or advertisers. Above all, they do not reduce the tax governments can derive from cigarette sales, and if tar content is reduced smokers hardly seem to notice. In the same month there were some minor adjustments to the tar tables – the amount of tar in what constituted low-tar, low- to middle-tar and middle-tar cigarettes was reduced slightly. Under the new system the maximum tar content allowed for low-tar cigarettes was set at 9 mg, compared with 10 mg under the old system. Under the new system low- to middle-tar cigarettes were to contain between 10 and 14 mg tar (as opposed to 11 to 16 mg under the old system), but the biggest change came in the high-tar brackets. Under the old system a cigarette was said to be high-tar if it contained 29 mg tar or more. Under the new system a cigarette counted as high-tar if it contained 18 mg tar or more and the old middle- to high-tar category, which covered cigarettes in the 23–8 mg tar range, was discontinued.

There have been many studies looking at the health effects of changing from high-tar to medium- and low-tar cigarettes. Certainly there is no doubt that such a change produces health benefits in terms of diseases of the lung but when it comes to assessing the health effects on other disorders like heart disease the comparison is not so easy. Smoking is only one of several important factors which contribute to the development of heart disease, and there is no evidence that deaths from coronary heart disease have been affected by the change from high-tar to low-tar cigarettes. There is also no evidence that the risks to babies and children of mothers who smoke are reduced by low-tar cigarettes. And as far as chest disorders go, the situation is clear.

Some studies looking at the health effects of changing to low-tar cigarettes have given equivocal results. A study carried out in Finland showed no real evidence that it was safer to smoke low-tar cigarettes yielding less than 10 mg tar than medium-tar cigarettes yielding between 10 and 18 mg. The survey found that young people aged sixteen to eighteen who smoked ten or more cigarettes a day were between two and a half and six times more likely to have respiratory symptoms compared with people who had never smoked, and there was little difference between smokers of low- and medium-tar cigarettes. The authors of the report said that low-tar cigarettes have a significant irritant effect on the lungs. In questioning why this should be so, the authors raised the issue of whether the tar yields as printed on the tar tables do indicate the real levels of tar being delivered to a smoker's lungs. They pointed out that the yields a smoker gets can be higher than the yields measured by standard laboratory methods, because the machines used to simulate smoking do not imitate the way a person smokes accurately. The result is that the real difference between low- and middle-tar cigarettes could be much smaller than imagined.

Firstly, there is the issue of compensatory smoking – people smoking low-tar cigarettes may smoke more of them, or smoke them more intensively, in order to get the effect they are used to. Some smokers puff harder and more often. But compensatory smoking may not altogether undo the benefits of switching to low-tar cigarettes. There is some evidence that compensatory smoking may increase the amount of nicotine and carbon monoxide getting into the body but not the tar. Then again, it has been suggested that if carbon monoxide is harmful to the heart, smoking filter cigarettes could actually increase the risk, as filter cigarettes in effect produce more carbon monoxide for the same nicotine yield.

A study carried out by the cigarette manufacturer Gallaher showed that, although there is some compensatory smoking, most smokers did receive less tar from smoking cigarettes in the low-tar category. The Gallaher researchers collected the cigarette butts from smokers over a twenty-four-hour period and estimated the smokers' tar intake from the amount of nicotine in the butts. They found that while smokers of low-tar cigarettes did partially compensate for the low nicotine level, 70 per cent had a mouth intake of tar which fell within or below the low-tar band. With middle-tar cigarettes 98 per cent of smokers had a tar intake by mouth which was within or below that stated on the label.

Whether compensatory smoking is significant or not, it is clear from looking at the figures for deaths among young smokers in the 1950s that the high-tar cigarettes then in general use did cause a much higher death toll than the cigarettes available now; the reduction in the death rate which has occurred since then can only be accounted for by the introduction of filter-tipped cigarettes and, more recently, of low-tar cigarettes. Thirty-eight men per million in the age group thirty to thirty-four died annually from lung cancer in the period 1951–5. By 1983 only ten men per million in this age range died from this disease – a reduction of 74 per cent. In the forty-five to forty-nine age group nearly 600 men per million died each year from 1951 to 1955. By 1983 the death rate in this age group had halved to 295 per million.

This reduction has not been paralleled in America and this could be because, while in Britain smoking stabilized among men in the 1940s, in America it increased rapidly between 1940 and 1960.

To return to the question of estimating tar yields per cigarette, there has been a great deal of discussion both by scientists and in the courts about the reliability of the testing methods. The issue is important to the tobacco industry because any success at cheating the tar tables – by making a cigarette which gives a low-tar reading on the tar tables yet which delivers more tar and nicotine to the smoker, giving it a 'fuller flavour' – could result in a sizeable segment of the market being captured and hence fat profits.

The official tar tables are produced from measurements on an automated smoking machine, which takes a 35 cc puff for two seconds once a minute until a standard butt is left. An article in the *New Scientist* traced the origin of testing cigarettes this way to work done in 1933 in America. This work involved tests on seven smokers who, it was found, puffed from 29 to 61 cc of smoke each time they drew on a cigarette. The robot smoker was originally produced as a way of testing Lucky Strike cigarettes, which were the most popular at the time. The *New Scientist* questioned whether this was the best method of testing cigarettes because, it pointed out, cigarettes have changed in both design and size and more recent research seems to show that smokers smoke very differently now than they did in the 1930s. The average puff lasts slightly longer than two seconds and draws in some 43 cc of smoke every 26 seconds. Yet the British machines still take a puff which is 20 per cent smaller, somewhat quicker and less than half as frequent. The *New Scientist* claimed that this meant that the official tar tables probably underestimated the amount of nicotine and tar the smoker takes in. These claims are denied by the Laboratory of the Government Chemist, which draws up the tar tables. Work to be published in late 1986 or early the following year will show that however cigarette brands are tested, their relative position in the tar tables remains by and large unchanged. The tests produce a ranking for cigarettes. Scientists involved in this work claim that even if a smoker smoked a low-tar cigarette particularly heavily he would still be unlikely to take in as much tar as he would if he smoked a brand from the next highest category normally.

There is another difference between the way a machine smokes and the way a human smokes, which, it has been claimed, has been exploited by one cigarette manufacturer to 'cheat' the tar tables. In America Brown & Williamson, a subsidiary of British American Tobacco, introduced a new type of filter in 1981. The 'Actron' filter seemed to be able to beat the smoking machine, giving readings for a lower tar content than that actually delivered. The filter has grooves running through it just underneath the paper wrapping. These grooves draw in air through holes in the side of the filter about half an inch from the end of the filter. In a smoking machine, which holds the cigarette gently by its end, Barclay cigarettes produce a 1 mg tar rating, but when these cigarettes are smoked by people, the grooves tend to be crushed by the smoker's fingers or lips, thus blocking the inflow of air which, in the machine, dilutes the smoke. Brown & Williamson strongly denies that its filter in any way cheats the tar tables.

Barclay cigarettes were advertised as being 99 per cent tar free, because they only contained 1 mg tar measured on the machine. It was a very successful advertising ploy. In 1983 Barclay cigarettes had a 1.3 per cent share of the American market, worth about £175 million a year.

BAT's competitors rumbled what was happening and complained to the Federal Trade Commission. A legal battle ensued, and eventually the Federal Trade Commission won. They made it clear that their testing method could not be relied on to promote the idea that the cigarette produced just 1 mg tar. Three independent scientific investigators appointed by the Federal Trade Commission maintained that the tar rating for Barclay cigarettes should be between 3 and 7 mg. By December 1983 BAT was forced to take down posters all over America advertising Barclay cigarettes as 99 per cent tar free, but by encouraging legal wrangling and by disputing the best way of measuring tar and nicotine content, BAT had bought time to consolidate Barclay's position in the market place.

Even though BAT had been prevented from making what were misleading advertising claims in America, it still went ahead with plans to make similar claims in other parts of the world. On 29 June 1984 the State Court in Geneva ordered the provisional seizure of all Barclay cigarette packets held by BAT which carried the 1 mg tar claim, and prohibited the company from using the claim in its advertising. BAT obtained a stay of the court order until the assertion that the Barclay filter 'deceived' cigarette-testing machines had been proved.

In Britain no attempt has been made to market this cigarette. The authorities say they are aware of the concern over the filter and would test it realistically if it ever became necessary.

At this time the tobacco companies were trying to develop substances which could be smoked like tobacco but which did not have undesirable ingredients. The Hunter Committee, consisting of an independent group of scientists, was set up in 1974 primarily to consider the scientific aspects of the use of tobacco substitutes and to be the final arbiter of whether these new substances were really less dangerous than cigarettes or not. The development of tobacco substitutes took several years, cost many millions of pounds and was an unmitigated disaster for the tobacco companies. They had hoped that they could produce a low-tar cigarette by literally diluting the tobacco with artificial substances which burned 'clean', that is without producing unpleasant and dangerous tar and nicotine.

There were several ventures. ICI in partnership with Imperial Tobacco spent some £20 million on one project. They built a factory in Ardeer in Scotland to produce their substitute, known as 'New Smoking Material'. Gallaher and Rothmans did something similar in partnership with the American Celanese Corporation and came up with a substance they called 'Cytrel'. After four years the Hunter Committee gave final approval to the product, saying that it 'may be no more dangerous to health than a similar product containing tobacco only and could prove to be less injurious'. It was an approval so cautious and qualified that it hardly amounted to any recommendation at all. Nevertheless the companies went ahead and marketed their new cigarettes. In fact most of the cigarettes contained only about 25 per cent tobacco substitute, the rest being ordinary tobacco. If the Hunter Committee had been noncommittal, the government was positively discouraging. In 1977 the then health minister, Roland Moyle, said, 'this is too serious a matter to mince words. Cigarettes with or without substitutes can be debilitating and ultimately lethal. For the government's part you can be assured that we will work relentlessly towards the ultimate object of a smoke-free society.'

The launch was a total flop. One year later the twelve brands containing tobacco substitute accounted for less than 1 per cent of the cigarette market and their production eventually stopped.

With the cloud hanging over cigarettes with or without substitutes some companies tried to expand on the tiny snuff market. Snuff had been popular in the days before machine-made cigarettes put tobacco within such easy reach of millions. Snuff is finely ground tobacco with various additives including salts, aromatics and flavourings. It was very popular in the seventeenth century. Tobacco manufacturers now saw this as a possible new way to interest people in tobacco. Health officials recognized that snuff-taking was probably very much safer than smoking, but it still carried a distinct risk of causing nasal cancer and they were not about to encourage its use as a smoking substitute.

Undaunted, one tobacco company blatantly set out to make snuff appealing to young people. Joseph and Henry Wilson of Sheffield, a subsidiary of Imperial Tobacco, placed an advertisement for snuff in the pop music newspaper *Melody Maker*, offering readers a free sample of 'refreshment at your fingertips'. The offer was supposedly restricted to people over eighteen years old, although it would have been difficult for the company to check whether those replying were over eighteen or not. The wording on the advertisement was designed to entice youngsters who might not have thought about taking snuff before. It read, 'Have you experienced the snuff sensation yet?' and went on, 'Wow, it's heady stuff. Well here's your chance to delight in the sensual pleasure of snuffing for free'. Those answering the advertisement received a free box of snuff and a booklet giving instructions on how to use it. Imperial Tobacco clearly saw a big future in the snuff business. In 1984 it paid out well over £3 million to acquire three snuff-manufacturing businesses, Conwood SA, Illingworth's of Kendal, Cumbria, and Wittman Gmbh of Konstanz, West Germany.

The way the tobacco industry marketed snuff took an alarming turn in the 1970s, when a new product was launched in America known as Skoal Bandits. These were tiny sachets of snuff rather like miniature tea bags, which were designed to be held in the mouth between the cheek or lip and the gum so that the tobacco got wet and the nicotine in it soaked out and entered the bloodstream through the thin membranes on the inside of the mouth. The habit has caught on in a big way. In America among the young it is considered very macho. Various groups in America like sportsmen and rodeo riders set a bad example by using Skoal Bandits, giving the product a special appeal to youngsters. It is estimated that some twenty-two million Americans use Skoal Bandits. Sales are up 60 per cent since 1978. Local surveys in places like Oregon, Oklahoma and Texas suggest that between 20 and 40 per cent of high-school boys are chewing, or 'dipping' as it is called, many of whom started before the age of thirteen. There is also some suggestion that teenagers start on Skoal Bandits and then move on to smoking once they are addicted to nicotine.

Skoal Bandits are considered a serious health risk. Dentists claim the habit causes gums to recede, the teeth become loose, the biting surfaces become abraded and tough white patches can occur on the gums and cheeks which can turn cancerous. It also seems to be more addictive than smoking. The constituent which is responsible for oral cancer is thought to be N-nitrosonornicotine, derived from the action of bacteria or enzymes on nicotine during curing. The nitrates in saliva seem to increase the quantities of N-nitrosonornicotine to levels much higher than those found in tobacco smoke.

The health hazards were brought home in a particularly stark way by just one case history – that of Sean Marsee, who started using Skoal Bandits when he picked up some free samples at a local rodeo. By the time he entered high school he was using seven to ten tins of the stuff a week. In 1983 he developed a sore on his tongue which would not heal. It was cancer. Over the next six months he had four operations in which he lost parts of his tongue, throat and jaw. He died in February 1984. He had been using Skoal Bandits for ten years. His case has become something of a *cause célèbre*, as his mother has now launched a multi-million dollar product-liability suit against the US Tobacco Company, which produces 90 per cent of the snuff 'tea bags' in America. The law suit claims that US Tobacco negligently and wrongly failed to place health warnings on the packets and that the product was promoted as a risk-free alternative to smoking.

The Federal Trade Commission has asked the US surgeon general to investigate the health hazards of 'snuff dipping'. There is little doubt that Skoal Bandits will be found to be harmful to health.

Despite the tragic consequences that snuff dipping is having in America the US Tobacco Company launched the same product on the British market in June 1984. Skoal Bandits were test-marketed in one small area at first; they were advertised over a ten-week period on Granada TV, in *TV Times* and in key local newspapers in the north west.

The company dismissed health fears about the product, despite claims that occasional users were four times and habitual users nearly fifty times more likely to develop oral cancer than those who did not use tobacco in any form. Yet astonishingly, there was apparently little the government could do, even if it wished to do anything. The government did negotiate a voluntary agreement with US Tobacco restricting the marketing of Skoal Bandits. Under the agreement, the company said it would refrain from marketing them to the under-eighteens or to non-smokers and it would also agree to limit the retail outlets. However, instead of being perceived by the public as a warning against the product, the company used the fact that it had concluded the agreement in such a way that, to the gullible, this could well be taken to imply government *approval* of the product. Mr Peter Parsons, a director of US Tobacco, wrote a letter to tobacconists on impressive headed notepaper, pointing out that the company had recently concluded a voluntary agreement with British health ministers, in which he said, 'in the light of this agreement we will continue to market Skoal Bandits in a positive and responsible manner'. The letter's discussion of the question of the safety of Skoal Bandits was even worse. The tobacco company once again fell back on the tired and much-criticized arguments the industry has used in the past to refute the evidence about the dangers of cigarette smoking. The letter said, 'The basic fact is that smokeless tobacco has not been scientifically established as a cause of any disease in humans, including oral cancer. To date no one knows the cause of oral cancer, nor can anyone explain the mechanism or mechanisms whereby this disease is caused.' He ended by saying what was needed was more research 'before any conclusions can be drawn'. Once again, the tobacco company was prevaricating while it presumably hoped an increasing number of young people would become hooked on smokeless tobacco, enabling it to build up a profitable business.

What upset the British Medical Association and anti-smoking organizations was not just that the government had done nothing to prevent the product being launched in Britain but that it had actually encouraged it by providing a grant to build a factory at East Kilbride in Scotland. Indeed, the company quickly realized that it had had an easy ride and was quoted as saying it had encountered 'surprisingly little opposition to its launch plans'.

In April 1985 the government's chief medical officer, Dr Donald Acheson, did write to all doctors warning of the dangers of Skoal Bandits and recommending that smokers who were tempted to try the sachets out as an alternative to smoking should consider other, safer ways of giving up. In December 1985 a Private Members' Bill was introduced in Parliament to make it illegal to sell tobacco products like Skoal Bandits to under sixteen-year-olds. It was introduced by the Labour MP for East Lothian, John Home Robertson. The BMA urged the government to encourage the enforcement of the bill's provisions.

Fighting the Giants

When the Royal College of Physicians first report, *Smoking and Health*, was published in 1962 it not only provided the first 'official' recognition of the fact that smoking was dangerous, it also triggered the creation of the anti-smoking lobby – seemingly a small voice crying in the wilderness initially, but a voice which has grown until today it is having major successes in changing attitudes and a modest success in reducing cigarette consumption. The 1962 report made many sweeping recommendations. It urged that there should be more imagination and effort put into warning the public about the dangers of tobacco. It wanted education aimed specifically at children and more effective restrictions on the sale of tobacco to children under sixteen. The regulation forbidding the sale of cigarettes to children was widely flouted and the report pointed out that cigarettes were widely available in slot machines. On advertising the report seemed to accept the cigarette manufacturers' claims that advertising did not do much to initiate the smoking habit and that it was designed to attract smokers to particular brands rather than to increase overall consumption. With hindsight it was a naïve view, but the report did call for legislation to restrict advertisements. It also called for much wider restrictions on smoking in public places, in an attempt to alter the social acceptability of the habit. It wanted heftier taxes on cigarettes and a reduction of taxation on cigar and pipe tobacco to persuade people to change to the less hazardous types of smoking. It wanted the tar content of cigarettes printed on the packet and experimental anti-smoking clinics set up in hospitals and chest clinics throughout the country.

The report made a substantial, if temporary, impact on cigarette consumption. Sales dropped sharply. But as the initial shock of the report's findings wore off, sales rose again to a figure only just below that in the year before the report was published.

The report also had some influence on government. In a voluntary agreement in 1962 British tobacco manufacturers accepted a code which was designed to exclude any cigarette advertisements which over-emphasized the pleasures of smoking, featured hero-figures, appealed to manliness, romance or social success or implied greater safety in any brand. Cigarette advertising on television was stopped in 1965. However, most of the report's recommendations were ignored.

Nine years later when the RCP published its second report on the subject, it was able to report only marginal progress. Although patterns of smoking among the population had changed slightly, the percentage of men who smoked had fallen only a little since 1962. There had been a slight decrease in smoking among men in professional and skilled occupations but there had been no change among men in social classes four and five. The percentage of women who smoked had declined slightly in social classes one to four but had risen in social class five – and those who did smoke were apparently smoking more. Once again, the 1971 report catalogued the dangers of smoking. It said that smoking was as important a cause of death as were the great epidemic diseases like typhoid, cholera and tuberculosis that had affected previous generations. It castigated the government for taking no effective action in the preceding nine years since the first report on smoking and health, even though it had accepted the evidence in that report that smoking was dangerous. The report described the death toll from smoking as 'a holocaust'.

Once again, it suggested a range of different projects to reduce the smoking habit and it went further. It urged the setting-up of a central smoking research unit, which would not only carry out much of the required research but would also co-operate with other groups of research workers in special fields, including those in the tobacco industry. It pointed out that the Medical Research Council had already set up various specialist research units and added, 'none could be of greater potential benefit to the country's health than one concerned with the problem of smoking and health'. The advice was ignored.

By 1977, when the RCP published its third report on the subject, its experts found themselves making many of the same points, but they widened their criticism to include the trade unions.

We regret that trade unions have so far shown no interest in the effects of smoking on the health of their members, while they devote close attention to smoking on the health of their members, while they devote close attention to industrial diseases, which now do incomparably less harm to working men's health than does smoking. We urge them to be more realistic.

Over the years, however, the message was making an impact. Education programmes had started and if government action had been half-hearted, others were taking up the cudgels. By 1983 and the fourth RCP report, smoking had been reduced but largely through voluntary effort. Once again, the report attacked the government for inaction, saying that legislation had been lacking and voluntary agreements with the tobacco industry had been largely ineffective.

However, there had been a shift in attitudes. The percentage of men smoking had fallen from 75 per cent in 1956 to 50 per cent in 1981. With women it was a different story. Between 1961 and 1976 the proportion of women smoking had remained constant at about 42 to 44 per cent. Both men and women were smoking fewer cigarettes. The number smoked by men had declined by some 20 per cent since the peak in 1960; the amount smoked by women had peaked in 1974 before declining.

Sales of tobacco in Britain had reached a record high in the early 1960s, when for three years they exceeded 270 million pounds in weight a year, but since 1974 they had been falling consistently in Britain, reaching 226 million pounds in 1981. The decline is only moderately encouraging, because 226 million pounds of tobacco still makes a very large number of cigarettes – and large numbers of both men and women continue to die from smoking-related diseases.

The fourth RCP report once again attacked the government.

The Royal College of Physicians would be failing in its duty if it did not urge the government to reverse its present attitude of inactivity and even of encouragement to the tobacco industry and tackle this hidden holocaust, with the urgency once given to cholera, diphtheria, poliomyelitis and tuberculosis.

The main difference between these infectious diseases and those caused by smoking, however, is that the government would lose a colossal amount of revenue were smoking ever to be abolished, so the motivation is not there. This was recognized publicly by the tobacco industry in a particularly cynical comment made by Dr Herbert Bentley, the managing director of Imperial Tobacco, in 1983. Worried about the possibility that the chancellor of the exchequer would the goose that lays the golden eggs'. In fact by increasing the tax on cigarettes the government would be doing just the opposite and increasing the size of the golden eggs.

Over the past twenty to thirty years the cost of cigarettes has actually come down in real terms. By February 1984 cigarettes were 40 per cent cheaper in real terms than they were in the 1950s.

The government had been nervous about putting up the tax on cigarettes as a way of discouraging smoking because, like Dr Bentley, it feared that fewer people would buy cigarettes as a result, and revenue would go down. In fact the government was also being too pessimistic. In 1984 Treasury estimates suggested that putting an extra 10p on the price of a packet of twenty cigarettes might put some people off buying cigarettes, but the net effect would be to increase tax revenues by some £320 million. A 25p increase would raise £765 million.

Following the Royal College of Physicians fourth report on smoking the *British Medical Journal* urged the Department of Health to produce a co-ordinated plan to tackle the problem. This would include a ban on advertising, changes in taxation, restriction on smoking in public places and at work and control of tobacco sponsorship of sport and culture. In a leading article it said the government 'has a responsibility to control smoking not only out of concern for the health of its own people but in full awareness of its exemplary role towards developing countries'.

The Times was also on the doctors' side. It accused the government of being too supine about discouraging smoking. It said that society was fully justified in restraining advertising where temptations were still so clever, pervasive and subtle, and also in ensuring that those who are offended by smoking need not suffer in public places. The *Lancet* focused on the report's findings on the dangers of passive smoking, or breathing other people's smoke, but suggested that this should not form a priority for medical research. It said far too much time, energy and money were being 'swallowed up by pointless research into the fine print of tobacco-related illness in smokers'. It also said the tobacco companies were too clever for the Department of Health in devising ways around the voluntary agreements on promotion.

The anti-smoking lobby has its friends in Parliament, but they are relatively few compared with those who see the freedom of the individual to smoke if he wants to as being more important than the freedom of the individual to walk in the street, travel by public transport and work in offices breathing clean air. One of the strongest anti-smoking speeches made in the House of Lords came from the patron of the anti-smoking organization, A S H (Action on Smoking and Health), in June 1984. This speech was of interest not only because of what it said but also because of who was making it – H R H the Duke of Gloucester. He condemned 'the indifference, ignorance and vested interest that continues to kill off that section of our society that cannot or will not save itself'. He pointed out that when the government health warning was introduced it seemed like a major advance. 'In retrospect it seems to have protected ethically and legally both the industry and government from the consequences of their action.' He called for a ban on the sponsorship of sports by the tobacco industry and said that succeeding generations would regard the issue of smoking with the same disdain the present generation now reserves for the policy and practice of slavery.

In the House of Commons the minority of MPs who want firmer action on smoking are outnumbered by the lobby which favours 'freedom'. The tobacco industry has considerable support in the House of Commons. When London Transport banned smoking on the underground an amendment to a motion congratulating London Transport on the ban said it deplored the decision to ban smoking in a minority of segregated compartments, on the grounds that London Transport has a duty to provide transport for the maximum number of potential customers while maximizing its return on capital. Its decision, said the amendment, 'can only reduce both usage and income'. It was a misleading amendment. One of its signatories was the former junior health minister, Sir Geoffrey Finsberg.

The government behaves paradoxically. On the one hand it acknowledges the damage smoking does and it supports organizations like the Health Education Council and Action on Smoking and Health. On the other hand it rewards tobacco companies which increase their sales. When Carreras Rothman won a Queen's Award for Export Achievement in 1983 A S H commented that to reward a company for exporting cigarettes 'was as sick as you can get', and compared it to giving a rabid dog a prize at Crufts.

The main thrust of Britain's anti-smoking campaign is now spearheaded by ASH, the Health Education Council (HEC) and the British Medical Association. ASH started life in 1971 with a grant of £13,000 from the government and an office lent by the Royal College of Physicians. By 1985 the government grant had increased to £150,000. The organization is now run from cramped offices in Mortimer Street, opposite the Middlesex Hospital in London. The HEC started in 1968, taking over from the Central Council for Health Education. Its role was general health education but in the 1970s it soon recognized that its main priority should be smoking, and that is still its most important priority. Twenty per cent of its annual budget of £10 million is devoted to it – much of it to anti-smoking advertising. The rest of its money is spent on things like educational programmes for schools, leaflets, support for GPs and also research.

Between 1980 and 1985 more than five million adults gave up smoking and the HEC claims some credit for this, partly by fostering a general change in the climate of opinion. However, it has not always been highly regarded by the medical profession. In 1982 a leading article in the *British Medical Journal* complained that ever since the Health Education Council started in 1968, it had never really got off the ground. The article suggested that one way of improving its effectiveness would be to respond brightly and quickly to media inquiries and to create news rather than merely reacting to it. It should hold regular briefings for MPs. In the *BMJ*'s words, 'It should sell the British people the joy of not smoking and living a healthier life style.' A pious aim, but one which is more difficult to achieve than might be thought. What the *BMJ* leader-writer may not have appreciated is that the HEC has to tread a careful path for fear of upsetting its political masters and so it does some of its work 'behind the scenes', engineering research and propaganda for which it deliberately seeks no credit.

The anti-smoking groups have worked together on a number of projects. In 1981 ASH, the HEC and the Scottish Health Education Group produced 'give up smoking' kits and a booklet for family doctors. This project was based on research which showed that a concerted campaign launched through GPs can have a reasonable success rate – 5 per cent gave up smoking with the help of a structured campaign, compared with less than 0.5 per cent of a group of smokers who did not receive the specialist help.[18]

The BBC has also co-operated with the anti-smoking groups in putting out programmes on how to give up smoking. A series of six programmes broadcast in 1982 on stopping smoking had an audience of eight million people and led to requests from 120,000 people for leaflets. It is believed that the programme helped a lot of people to give up.

In 1985 the government, recognizing that the smoking habits of women were of particular concern, gave the Health Education Council an extra half a million pounds towards a campaign aimed particularly at women.

After years of disapproving of smoking from the sidelines, the British Medical Association decided in 1984 to launch its own campaign. Its track record for winning campaigns is good. It admits that it takes time, but two previous campaigns – against drinking and driving and in favour of seat-belt legislation – have eventually borne fruit, with impressive results in terms of lives saved.

The BMA anti-smoking campaign is aimed at stopping tobacco advertising and the promotion of cigarettes through sponsorship (see Chapter 10). The secretary of the BMA, Dr John Havard, described the existing voluntary agreement governing advertising and sports sponsorship as 'a farce' and 'a sick joke'. He made it clear it was time for doctors to speak out against tobacco promotion or, in his words, 'be guilty of collusion ... Every day we delay in banning the promotional activities of the industry, an average 274 premature deaths occur.'[19] He accused the tobacco companies of a massive cover-up exercise carried out world-wide by an industry which callously ignored the medical facts, and said, 'A young adult cannot pick up a magazine, read a newspaper, watch the television, or walk in the street without being bombarded by the tobacco industry. That is not freedom of choice – that is coercion.'

The launch of the BMA's own campaign was supported in a poignant letter from a newsagent writing in the trade paper, the *Newsagent*. He was himself a lung-cancer victim and he urged fellow newsagents 'in the name of humanity' to think of diversifying into other product areas before they forge ahead with any more cigarettes. He died shortly after writing the letter.

The tobacco industry fought back against the BMA, saying there was no evidence that there was any link between advertising and young people starting to smoke, a claim dismissed by Dr Havard as 'pathetic'.

As part of its campaign the BMA gave doctors a supply of black-edged postcards, which each doctor was asked to send to his MP every time a patient of his died from a disease caused by smoking. The cards read, 'I wish to inform you that one of your constituents who was a patient of mine has died. The death was due to the following disease ...' There followed a list of the three main illnesses caused by smoking, namely lung cancer, chronic obstructive lung disease and coronary heart disease, plus 'other related cancer or vascular diseases'. It went on, 'This person smoked. Tobacco smoking is the major avoidable cause of this disease.' Ten thousand cards were printed. If the death of every patient who died of a smoking-related disease had been notified to an MP in this way, the cards would have lasted a mere forty days.

It was an effective way of bringing the message home to MPs. Indeed, so effective was it that one MP became riled by what he saw as an unethical way of carrying on and set out to make an issue of it. The MP was Sir William van Straubenzee. He wrote to one doctor who had sent him one of these cards saying, 'you have chosen a particularly ghoulish method of informing me of a constituent's death. In order that I may investigate the matter carefully, I now call on you to give me the name and address of the constituent concerned.'

Such a disclosure would have been against medical ethics and despite several attempts by 'Sir Bill', as the local newspaper called him, the doctor refused to make any such disclosure. Reporting the MP's attempt to find out the constituent's name, one local paper quoted him as saying, 'I will hunt Dr Ingram. I will make life very troublesome for him, even if I have to draw attention to him through Parliament.' The MP made something of a fool of himself by claiming medical knowledge he clearly did not have, when he was quoted in the paper as saying that the biggest single killer disease was obesity and asserting that tobacco advertising was comparable to the advertising of sweets and cakes. The doctor's local colleagues invited

Sir William to come to their hospital to see the effects of smoking in their patients. He refused and was quoted as saying that when he was in charge of Northern Ireland's medical services, he had visited hospitals frequently, where he saw every kind of condition and illness. 'I have probably seen more of it than they have.' Then in another move which defies logic, he announced that he had reported the doctor to the General Medical Council for alleged breach of confidentiality! The GMC quickly dismissed the complaint.

The doctor was finally let down in his battle with the MP by his own health authority, which intervened and requested that the black-edged cards should not be sent with the hospital's name on them. It also wrote to the MP apologizing for the fact that he had apparently received another card. Writing about the saga in the *British Medical Journal*, the doctor concluded, 'this was particularly sad coming from a body with the responsibility of maintaining the health of the local population'.

In May 1985 the British Medical Association made it clear that it wanted to widen its campaign to make it world-wide. It called for an effective international organization to co-ordinate an attack on tobacco. Like infectious diseases, tobacco is a supra-national problem needing international co-operation to fight it. This was not the first time a call for international action had been made. In 1978 the European health ministers proposed an advisory committee on public health. At about the same time a similar idea was suggested by the BMA to the then president of the Commission, Roy Jenkins, but nothing was done.

The World Health Organization is one international body which has been active in campaigning against smoking. Its 1979 report on controlling the smoking epidemic recommended a total prohibition of all forms of tobacco promotion. One of its most recent initiatives was a campaign launched in association with the International Olympic Committee called 'Winners for Health'. It is aimed particularly at the Third World and its main target is the young – those aged twelve to twenty-five. The programme will include the use of major international and national sporting events to publicize important health messages, and the development of a range of international material for sport and health education.

If the British government has been acting illogically in tackling smoking – wringing its hands over the ill-effects while gathering in the revenue from the sale of cigarettes – then the American government finds itself in even more of a dilemma. Not only does it rely on the sale of tobacco to produce $25 billion of revenue, but also large sections of many states are devoted entirely to growing tobacco and producing cigarettes. Thousands of farms depend on the industry, as do some two million jobs. When the American surgeon general, Dr Everett Koop, called for a smoke-free society by the year 2000 in a speech at the annual meeting of the American Lung Association in May 1984, some politicians demanded his removal by the president.

Throughout the developed world the anti-smoking lobby is having a definite impact. Public attitudes are changing and legislation is being brought in to make it easier for people to avoid smoke. In London smoking was banned in underground trains in July 1984 and the following December smoking was banned in underground stations as well. In Australia all government offices have restrictions on smoking. In many American cities local by-laws now restrict smoking at work. Safety warnings on the cigarette packets have been tightened up in the United States. In September 1984 Congress finally gave approval for four new health warnings, each 50 per cent larger than the existing message. One warning points out that smoking 'causes lung cancer, heart disease, emphysema and may complicate pregnancy'. Another says, 'quitting smoking now greatly reduces serious risks to your health'.

The situation is improving elsewhere. In Russia smoking was banned on Aeroflot's domestic routes in 1983 and other airlines in the West are considering similar moves. Also in Russia, smoking is banned in public places including the cinema and the underground. Information campaigns in the media are thought to have helped to cause the decline in smoking in France, where the proportion of those who smoke has fallen from 44 per cent of the population in 1976 to 37 per cent in March 1982. In Iceland anti-smoking laws now force manufacturers to put not only a health warning on their packets but also one of six pictures: black lungs, a patient in bed, a pregnant mother, a diseased heart and coronary arteries, an inflamed nose and throat, or young children. In addition the law prohibits shops from displaying tobacco products. In Greece a two-year aggressive anti-smoking campaign stopped short the rise in cigarette consumption. The campaign included such things as anti-smoking advertisements on television, health warnings on all matchboxes and a campaign in schools and health centres.

One recent development in the war against the cigarette promoters has been the appearance of a number of organizations dedicated to making themselves a nuisance to the tobacco industry – a goal achieved by demonstrations and especially by defacing billboards and posters advertising cigarettes. The campaign started in Australia in the late 1970s, when an irreverently named organization, BUGA UP, made its presence felt on the city streets. BUGA UP is short for Billboard Utilizing Graffitists Against Unhealthy Promotions. Cleverly organized, it has had a public profile out of all proportion to the number of its activists and to its costs. Indeed its costs have been minimal – just the price of an aerosol can in many cases. Yet it has become a thorn in the side of the advertising industry and has managed to turn cigarette advertisements to its advantage in a way which has infuriated the cigarette manufacturers. For example, with a few deft strokes of the aerosol can a poster saying, 'New, mild and Marlboro' becomes 'New, Vile and a Bore'. An advertisement for Benson and Hedges featuring a chess game was changed by the addition of the words along the bottom 'have a lung check mate'. Dunhill becomes 'Lung Ill' and so on.

In Sydney, BUGA UP set up an 'embassy' outside the Leo Burnett advertising agency – one of the agency's clients is Philip Morris, which makes brands such as Marlboro, Peter Jackson, Alpine and Chesterfields. BUGA UP parked a caravan outside and distributed pamphlets. The Advertising Federation of Australia released a statement which it had sent to the premier of New South Wales, claiming that the 'embassy' was 'producing a media event and vilifying the agency by sight and sound for allegedly contributing to anti-social activity and endeavouring to suborn employees'. It also condemned BUGA UP for openly encouraging vandalism, apparently failing to see the irony that cigarette manufacturers themselves are openly encouraging people to kill themselves by smoking.

By October 1984 there had been twenty arrests of the graffitists, who included a general practitioner, an ear-nose-and-throat consultant, a radiologist, a paediatric renal physician, an occupational health physician and two medical students. Some were found guilty and given a minimum fine, some were released with a warning and others were acquitted. Their object was achieved, however: all the cases received massive publicity. Their defence was that their acts were committed to prevent a greater evil.

The success of BUGA UP in bringing the anti-smoking message to the notice of the public and the cigarette companies led to other similar organizations springing up in other countries. In Britain it spawned AGHAST (Action Group to Halt Advertising and Sponsorship by Tobacco). The organization's activities have included, for example, demonstrations against the National Theatre production of 'Tales from Hollywood' at a Bristol theatre, which was sponsored by John Player. AGHAST handed out leaflets advertising its version of the play – a parody entitled 'Tales from Hospital', which it described as 'a fascinating tale about the evil tobacco baron John Slayer, who masquerades as a philanthropist by sponsoring a National Theatre troupe. However, it soon becomes clear that this callous Slayer is little more than a drug pusher.'

Sir Peter Hall, the director of the National Theatre, reacted by hiding behind the skirts of the government, claiming that it was government policy that the theatre should get as much money as possible from sponsorship and adding that 'the tobacco industry, which is generous towards the arts, cannot be dismissed'. He added, 'The government itself earns a lot of money out of smoking.'

Anti-smoking propagandists in Britain have also been active with the aerosol can. One advertisement showing animal footprints in the snow with a cigarette packet nearly bitten through and bearing teeth marks was 'adjusted' by a can sprayer who added the words, 'Cancer bites back.'

Members of AGHAST have also demonstrated against other promotional activities like the Marlboro Adventure Travel Holidays. On one occasion they stood outside the branch of Thomas Cook in Bristol, trying to attract people to book up for their Ultimate Marblerow Holidays' – a reference to a row of marble tomb stones. Their 'promotional material' claimed that 'most of our holidays are as unashamedly removed from the uniformity and humdrum of today's life as gasping for breath in an oxygen mask is from breathing fresh air into healthy lungs'. The idea was to show 'where Marlboro cigarettes would really take you'.

Other organizations have adopted similarly imaginative acronyms like COGHIN (short for Citizens' Organization using Graffiti for Health in the Neighbourhood), and TREES (short for Those Resisting an Early End from Smoking). The latter is a group of doctors and nurses who say they are no longer prepared to sit by helplessly and watch people dying of tobacco-related diseases. One of their first stunts was to hand out sun visors at the 1985 final of the Benson and Hedges Cup at Lords, with the slogan 'B and H stumps your growth.' A large banner reading 'Kingsize Killers' was hung from the top of a building easily visible from the ground. TREES has protested vigorously against sponsorship of sport and the arts. At one ballet performance sponsored by John Player the organization's leaflets said that the sponsoring company's lethal products were being associated with images far removed from the ghastly realities of lung cancer, chronic bronchitis and early heart attacks. It accused the tobacco companies of being 'engineers of marketing schemes to addict hundreds of thousands of young people each year to a product which will kill 250 out of 1,000 smokers before their time'. They had recruited an impressive imaginary cast to take part in their 'dance of death', including Nick O'Teen, Bron Kytis and Magot Emphysema.

Irritating though these impromptu anti-smoking organizations are to the industry, they have recently been superseded by a potentially much more threatening group of professionals, which for the first time is beginning to have the tobacco barons trembling in their shoes. Three Texas law firms announced in March 1985 that they had formed a new state-wide organization of trial lawyers to deal exclusively with litigation based on diseases attributed to cigarette smoking. Lawyers in the so-called VigLit group will try to get the Texas courts to determine whether cigarette manufacturers can be held legally responsible for their disease victims. They argue that the manufacturers have suppressed the issuing of effective warnings on the nature and magnitude of the health dangers of smoking. They claim smoking is an addiction, not a voluntary activity, and the companies depend for their future wealth on seducing American children into addiction.

Already in November a US federal court judge, H. Lee Sarokin, had ruled that health warnings on cigarette packets did not debar smokers who had developed lung cancer from bringing law suits against tobacco companies. He said that the health warning, like many government standards, was meant to fix a minimum level of industry performance, but that 'legal minimums were never intended to supplant moral maximums'. He added that if Congress had intended that cigarette manufacturers could not be held liable in court they could have incorporated such language into the statute. He went on, 'before this court or any court so cavalierly rejects fundamental principles of the common law it should demand a much more definitive statement from Congress'.

His judgement marked another step in the attempt by a 58-year-old lung-cancer victim, Rose Cipollone, to claim damages for her illness from the manufacturers of the cigarette brands she smoked for forty years: Ligget Incorporated, a subsidiary of Grand Metropolitan, Philip Morris Incorporated and Lorillard.

In America there are now about forty-five product-liability suits awaiting trial. The cases are being brought by the families of dead or dying smokers on their behalf. The lawsuits rely on recent changes in the law and public attitudes to smoking, together with increasing scientific evidence linking smoking with lung cancer.

In the past American courts tended to take the view that smokers voluntarily assumed the risks of tobacco and that the companies could not be held liable when there was doubt about the link between smoking and lung cancer. However, now that there is a new awareness of the dangers of smoking, the anti-smoking lobby believes it is a good time to step up its legal campaign.

The situation became even more worrying for the tobacco companies in October 1985 when a former asbestos manufacturer, the GAF Corporation, filed 200 cross-complaints against the tobacco companies, claiming they should share the costs of any judgements in asbestos-liability cases because smoking can dramatically increase the risks of asbestos.

8. Smoking: The Government's Dilemma

Queen Elizabeth I was the first person to realize that a tax on tobacco could produce a tidy revenue for the exchequer and began a trend in the sixteenth century which now provides enough money to pay for a third of Britain's health service.

The first sovereign to despise tobacco and be in a position to do something about it was James I. To discourage smoking he increased the tax on tobacco by 4,000 per cent, from 2d. a pound to 6s. 8d. a pound. It worked too well: it had the desired effect of putting people off tobacco, but it also meant his revenue was cut, so he reduced the tax to just 2s. a pound.

The revenue from tobacco tax has been the most important reason why governments have failed to take effective action against the tobacco companies, even though some have explained their lack of aggressive action by saying that they did not want to interfere with the basic freedom of the individual to choose to smoke if he wants to or of tobacco companies to market a legal product.

Doctors have for a long time urged increases in tobacco tax as a way of discouraging smoking. In 1971 the second report by the Royal College of Physicians recommended similar action, although it did draw attention to the difficulties this might cause for addicted smokers on a small income. It was worried they might be so habituated that they would continue to smoke and have less money for essential family needs. Rather quaintly, the report also mentioned the possibility that more expensive cigarettes might lead to increases in crime. 'Lorry loads of cigarettes already provide a tempting bait for criminals, and the more expensive the cigarettes the more tempting they would be.'

This report also urged that there should be an official inquiry into the economic consequences of a decrease in cigarette smoking and that a full report showing the balance of benefit and loss be published.

The investigation was carried out, but a full report was never published, at least not officially – many years later the inquiry's findings were leaked to the *Guardian* and appeared on 6 May 1980. The study was completed by a group of senior officials from various government departments chaired by someone from the Cabinet Office. They found that if there were no reduction in smoking, an estimated one and a half million people would die prematurely by the year 2000. A 20 per cent reduction over a thirty-year period ending in the year 2000 would mean a quarter of a million lives would be saved, a 40 per cent drop would save half a million lives over the same period. There would also be a considerable fall in the number of people losing time off work through sickness caused by smoking.

The disadvantage from the cost point of view would be that although health-care costs would be saved in the short term, people would live longer, so there would be more retired people, representing an increased drain on the resources of the Department of Health and Social Security. In financial terms a 20 per cent fall in smoking would save the government £4 million in health-care costs by 1981, but increased social security costs would amount to an extra £12 million by the year 2000. A 40 per cent drop in smoking would cost the government an extra £29 million by the end of the century. These costs would be much higher now when measured in 1986 pounds.

The report also showed there would also be a net fall in the revenue from cigarettes. Although people would spend their money on other things, the tax on cigarettes was so high that it would be difficult to replace it without imposing very much higher taxes elsewhere. A reduction of 20 per cent in the sale of cigarettes would result in a loss of £150 million by 1981. A 40 per cent drop would lose the government £305 million. There would also be a cost in increased unemployment as cigarette factories closed. To make matters worse, the unemployment would occur in areas where unemployment was already high: Northern Ireland, Scotland and the north east. With tobacco revenue raising some £1 billion a year, it was no wonder that a former minister of health, Ian MacLeod, said, 'smokers, mainly cigarette smokers, contribute some £1,000 million yearly to the exchequer and no one knows better than the government that it simply cannot afford to lose that much'.

As the full report on the economics of smoking was not published at the time the study was carried out, a feeling remained among doctors that increasing the price of cigarettes to cut consumption would be financially beneficial. The 1977 Royal College of Physicians report *Smoking or Health* said that although it was difficult to draw up a balance sheet, 'our conclusion is that the overall financial consequences of any reduction in smoking which is likely to occur in this generation will be favourable'.

Whether it was fear of losing revenue or not, it now seems odd that between 1947 and 1974 tobacco tax was not significantly increased. By the early seventies cigarettes had become relatively cheaper than they were in the 1950s, when their danger was first realized. A historic first occurred in 1975 when the chancellor of the exchequer, Denis Healey, said in his budget speech that he had increased tax differentially on cigarettes in order to discourage their sale, something his predecessors had said was impossible to do. In the three years 1974–6, tax increases raised the price of a packet of twenty cigarettes by 5 per cent. This alarmed the cigarette manufacturers. After the 1976 price increase some of them held their prices down for a while to maintain their sales. In December 1976 a further 10 per cent price increase was added. The tax increases in the mid-seventies marked the beginning of the decline in cigarette sales, which had reached their peak in 1973, when over 137 billion cigarettes were sold in Britain. By 1980 sales had fallen to 120 billion.

In 1981 the tax on cigarettes was increased twice, making the price of a packet of twenty cigarettes £1.00. Cigarette sales dropped ten billion, which meant that the tobacco industry had to shed jobs. However, sales did not fall as much as some had predicted. The irony of it was that despite the fall in sales, the government actually made more money. From this experience and similar findings in other countries, it seemed that a 10 per cent increase in price actually produced a decrease of 5 per cent in sales. If maintained, this would imply a saving of about 5,000 lives a year.

By 1981 the tobacco industry had become acutely worried about what was happening and the pressure they were experiencing. They carried out their own economic study and produced a report entitled *The UK Tobacco Industry – Its Economic Significance*. This pointed out that the tobacco industry provided £4 billion of government revenue, 35,000 manufacturing jobs, and 265,000 jobs overall; it accounted for a tobacco trade surplus of £245 million on the balance of payments and consumer spending of £4.8 billion – nearly 4 per cent of all the money people spend in Britain.

However, sales still fell. The industry's warnings had little effect. By 1983 sales had fallen by as much as a quarter compared to the peak ten years earlier. By 1983 too, smoking had become a party-political issue, though with varying degrees of commitment. None of the parties were too sure as yet exactly how many votes there were in being anti-smoking.

The Labour Party's manifesto for the general election that year made a vague reference to tobacco, saying it would 'act' on cigarette advertising, without saying what it intended to do. This vague commitment was said to be a compromise, because the unions claimed that any action against cigarettes would result in lost jobs. According to one commentator, 'the economic argument has therefore taken precedence in the Labour Party over moral and medical imperatives'.[20]

The Social Democrats claiming to be keen to cut smoking promised to reduce 'substantially' the promotion of tobacco. The SDP also proposed to bring tobacco under the Medicines Act. It believed that this would provide a mechanism for the detailed evaluation of the effects of tobacco products. It would also allow regulations to be laid down to control tobacco more carefully. The evaluation of the effects of tobacco products has been fully documented already.

Mr Norman Tebbit, for the Conservatives, clearly did not support an anti-smoking stance. Then employment minister, he told workers at a Carreras Rothman factory that the Conservatives did not want to see cigarette advertising stopped, although they would continue to issue health warnings so that people could make up their own minds about smoking. He said, 'if we give in to the people who want to stop smoking, then we will have to give in to those people who want to stop drinking, or taking sugar in tea because it is fattening, or skiing because it is supposedly dangerous'. The government is apparently willing to listen to those people who quite rightly want to stop the peddling of heroin to youngsters because of its undoubted dangers, but is less concerned about the peddling of cigarettes to youngsters, which causes 1,000 times as many deaths, although admittedly later in life. And whoever said that taking sugar in tea or having the occasional drink was dangerous?

The tobacco industry continued to worry about the effect that a big rise in tobacco tax could have on sales. In one advertisement it warned that should the government be deprived of tobacco tax then there could be a big rise in VAT. The advertisement hit home with one *Guardian* reader, but not in the way the tobacco industry hoped. The reader wrote to the *Guardian*: 'having spent most of 1982 in hospital, I have just come home for a short respite after my tenth operation – a series of endeavours by the surgeons to lessen the damage of cancer. I now know that I shall never be able to converse or eat normally again. Perhaps the Tobacco Advisory Council could advise me what I should do with my new-found knowledge about VAT.'

The March 1984 budget once again loaded tax on tobacco products. The government maintained its policy of increasing tax at a higher rate than inflation. It no longer seemed such an anti-social or unpopular thing to do. The tax on a packet of twenty cigarettes was raised by 10p and there were similar increases on hand-rolled tobacco. Predictably, the industry squealed. It said it was 'stunned' by the increase, which was 'harsh and unfair'. The newsagents' trade publication claimed that the Treasury would actually lose revenue as a result of this tax increase. Independent experts thought otherwise. A tobacco analyst at a large stockbroker estimated that even if consumption declined by 4 or 5 per cent, the Treasury would gain about £250 million.

In fact a series of estimates by the Treasury in December 1984 showed that the government could probably increase the tax on cigarettes considerably more without fear of losing revenue. They estimated that a further 10p rise on a packet of twenty would produce some £320 million in revenue in a full year; a 20p increase would increase revenue by £625 million and a 25p increase would produce a staggering £770 million in revenue, despite the fact that the higher prices would undoubtedly put a lot of people off smoking. The Treasury did admit, however, that the estimates were subject to considerable uncertainty for the larger price increases. Ironically, some of the money the government raised in taxes was in fact used to feed 'the goose which lays the golden egg'. Between April 1979 and January 1985 the British government gave over £5 million in selective assistance to several tobacco companies, including Carreras Rothman Limited, Imperial Tobacco Limited and J. R. Freeman and Son Limited.

By the March 1985 budget the government was ready once again to increase the tax on cigarettes by more than inflation: 6p went on a packet of twenty. An inflation-linked increase would have meant an increase of just about half that amount. The increase was expected to yield an additional £180 million in a full year. According to one tobacco analyst, it would lead to a 3 per cent drop in consumption. In the 1986 budget the tax on a packet of twenty cigarettes was increased by 11p – once again well above the inflation rate, but there were no increases on pipe tobacco or cigars.

The government's commitment to stopping people smoking has always been half-hearted. One of the clearest signs of this came in 1983, when the Royal College of Physicians fourth report on smoking and health, *Health or Smoking*, was produced. On the very day this report was published the health ministers met FOREST, the organization set up by the tobacco industry to lobby for their cause. At about this time the Department of Health also blocked the appointment of a former director of ASH, Mike Daube, to a post at the Health Education Council for which he seemed the most obvious candidate. It was suggested at the time that this could have been because he had used some intemperate words at a recent conference on smoking – he had reportedly called the tobacco manufacturers mass murderers – and it was felt the industry would balk at having to co-operate with such a person at the HEC. In fact later evidence showed he did not use those words. There was also evidence that the industry had itself lobbied against his appointment. The government was apparently keen for the Health Education Council to co-operate more closely with the tobacco industry, although it was never quite clear to what purpose. Mr Kenneth Clarke, the health minister at the time, reportedly wrote to the chairman of the HEC, Sir Brian Bailey, saying he hoped Sir Brian would be able to involve the council with industrial interests on an increasing scale. He also said in his letter that he noted the decline in male lung-cancer mortality 'since the tobacco industry embarked on their programme to reduce the tar delivery of cigarettes'. It was a letter regarded by many in the health-education field as crass. The political editor of the *Observer*, Adam Raphael, wrote that he thought the letter bordered on the improper. 'Health ministers should not be promoting the interests of the tobacco manufacturers,' he said.

Following the publication of the Royal College of Physicians fourth report the government was asked in the House of Lords what action it intended to take. Lord Glenarthur said the government was committed to do all it could to discourage smoking and so reduce the deaths, disease and illness associated with it, but he added that he could not accept that all the criticisms made by the report were necessarily justified. He said one had to be very careful about imposing a ban on advertising in a free society unless there was firm evidence to support one. He said that in this case there was no clear evidence that a ban on advertising would affect overall consumption, and anyway there did not seem to be majority support for such a ban in the community.

In the history of the relationship between Western governments and the tobacco industry, the stories of two people, both at one time government ministers, illustrate in the clearest possible way the strength of the tobacco lobby and the difficulty anti-smoking organizations face when trying to tackle an issue where there are such huge vested interests. One is the case of Sir George Young, a junior health minister in the Thatcher government of 1979; the other is that of Joe Califano, secretary of state for Health and Welfare in President Carter's government.[21]

To take the case of Sir George Young first. Of all the health ministers Britain has had, he was the most committed in the fight against the tobacco barons, and the industry recognized and feared this. One of the first things the industry did to counteract his zeal was to set up the front organization FOREST – the Freedom Organization for the Right to Enjoy Smoking Tobacco. This was a particularly unfortunate acronym, as the tobacco industry has done a great deal to destroy much of the Third World's forests, as we shall see in Chapter 12. It was the idea of its chairman, a former Battle of Britain fighter pilot and commander-in-chief of RAF Germany, Air Chief Marshall Sir Christopher Foxley-Norris.

The organization was launched on 18 June 1979, when Sir George Young and most of the anti-smoking lobby were in Stockholm at the fourth World Conference on Smoking and Health. Foxley-Norris soon learned the jargon of the industry; when challenged on the health aspects of smoking he trotted out what has come to be the industry's stock answer: 'we are medically unqualified to comment or make judgement'.

In December 1979 negotiations began for a new agreement between the Department of Health and the tobacco industry. The Department of Health shopping list made it clear to the industry that Sir George Young and his secretary of state, Patrick Jenkin, meant business. The Department of Health wanted an end to all poster and cinema advertising and a 50 per cent reduction in all other advertising. It also wanted a new health warning. The industry was shocked. One of their claims had always been that they were not interested in selling to young people, but half way through the negotiations the industry's lies were exposed in a most fortuitous way. Sir George Young revealed that the young son of his official driver had received on his eighteenth birthday an unsolicited invitation through the post to join Philip Morris's Club Marlboro in return for ten Marlboro packet tops. The inducement to smoke was clear. Once he joined he would be entitled to free or half-price entry to dozens of UK clubs and discos. He would get albums and tapes at cheap prices and special terms on tickets to Brands Hatch or Silverstone race meetings. On top of this there would be discounts on sports and hi-fi equipment and information on how to learn skiing, hang-gliding, etc. In fact he was a non-smoker.

The pressure on the tobacco industry was such that after negotiations lasting twelve months they agreed to a compromise, because they feared that unless they did so there could well be legislation. Under the new agreement there would be a 30 per cent cut in poster advertising, a series of new warnings – 'Most doctors don't smoke' was one – and restrictions on promotions. In addition, the industry agreed to provide £1 million for research into the effects of low-tar cigarettes. The agreement was to last for twenty months. Patrick Jenkin and Sir George Young then decided that when the twenty-month period was over they should use legislation to bring in the restrictions they could not get through voluntary agreement. It was clear they meant business. In the event, there was a shortage of parliamentary time and the plans did not come to anything.

Meanwhile, the agreement on sports sponsorship negotiated by the sports minister in the Department of the Environment in 1977 was due to expire in 1980 but had been extended for a further year because Sir George did not want to see a soft agreement on sport while he was trying to get legislation through Parliament. Patrick Jenkin tried to persuade the then sports minister, Hector Monro, that there was a need for a tougher agreement, and an especial need to remove the brand names from the title of sports events. This would mean for example, that the Benson and Hedges Cup would be the Gallaher's Cup, and the John Player League would become the Imperial League. But Patrick Jenkin did not get his way, and Sir George Young was just as unsuccessful.

The industry was becoming increasingly concerned about the activities of Sir George Young and used all its muscle to get him moved. It did not have to wait long. In 1981 Mrs Thatcher moved him to the Department of the Environment. Patrick Jenkin was promoted to the Department of Industry and Norman Fowler replaced him as social services secretary.

The following year a sports sponsorship agreement was finally signed by the new sports minister, Neil Macfarlane. Later a new voluntary agreement was reached between the tobacco industry and the new health ministers – health warnings were changed back to the old weaker one, 'Warning: cigarettes can seriously damage your health'. The size of the warnings was increased and the industry was to give £11 million over the course of the agreement for health-promotion research, especially among young people. This latest quasi-philanthropic gesture by the industry was not what it seemed, as the conditions imposed upon it meant that the money could not be used 'directly or indirectly to examine the use and effects of tobacco products' (see Chapter 10).

The other government minister to flex his muscles over the smoking issue, only to find that they were clearly weaker than the collective muscle of the tobacco industry's lobbyists, was Joe Califano, health secretary in President Carter's government. He warned America that smoking was 'slow-motion suicide'. He was struck by two things: first, 90 per cent of adult smokers had tried to give it up within the previous twelve months, and second, 75 per cent of smokers were hooked before they were twenty-one. However, his anti-smoking zeal began to worry President Carter's advisers. Califano's anti-smoking programme was launched in a blaze of publicity and labelled cigarette smoking 'public enemy number one'. He pointed out that cigarettes killed 320,000 Americans every year, 220,000 from heart disease and 22,000 from respiratory diseases. His campaign began to spell trouble for President Carter. Three times Carter visited North Carolina, the place he termed the 'greatest tobacco-producing state in the world'. He assured the people there he was committed to a balanced campaign to protect the health of the tobacco industry.

Meanwhile, in 1979 Califano commissioned a special surgeon general's report to mark the fifteenth anniversary of the first report in 1964. In his introduction Califano wrote that the report 'demolishes the claims made by cigarette manufacturers and a few others fifteen years ago and today that the scientific evidence was sketchy and that no link between smoking and cancer was proven. Those claims, empty then, are utterly vacuous now.' The report contained more disturbing statistics. For example, the percentage of girls who smoked had increased eightfold since 1968. Among the age group thirteen to nineteen there were now six million regular smokers. It also said that 100,000 children under thirteen were regular smokers. In the two weeks after its publication more Americans tried to give up smoking than in any other two-week period since the first surgeon general's report was published in 1964.

Califano went to the fourth World Conference on Smoking and Health in June 1979, where he told the delegates that the surgeon general had summarized '... the decisive and devastating evidence added in the past fifteen years [which convicts] cigarette smoking beyond a reasonable doubt of crimes against public health'. Soon after he got back Califano was fired. He had been President Carter's health secretary for two and a half years – about the same length of time that Sir George Young lasted as a junior health minister in Mrs Thatcher's government.

During President Reagan's election campaign, there was a lot of fence mending to do. Reagan made his position clear in a letter to a farmer in Greenville, North Carolina, in the heart of the tobacco country. In it he said, 'I can guarantee that my own cabinet members will be far too busy with substantive matters to waste their time proselytizing against the dangers of cigarette smoking.'

Reagan's new health team commissioned yet another report from the surgeon general. It was published in 1982 as part of the continuing series *The Health Consequences of Smoking*. The surgeon general, Dr Everett Koop, said in his introduction that cigarette smoking was 'the chief, single avoidable cause of death in our society and the most important public health issue of our time'.

Reagan's commitment not to waste time proselytizing against cancer was thrown back at him many times during his presidency whenever tobacco interests feared they were under threat from his government. In May 1984 a new agreement was reached on health warnings on cigarette packets sold in America. Up until then the warning had been simply, 'The surgeon general has determined that cigarette smoking is dangerous to your health'. Now one of the following sentences was to be printed under the heading 'Surgeon General's Warning': 'Smoking causes lung cancer, heart disease, emphysema and may complicate pregnancy'; 'Quitting smoking now greatly reduces serious risk to your health'; 'Smoking by pregnant women may result in foetal injury, premature birth and low birth weight'; or 'Cigarette smoke contains carbon monoxide'.

In many ways any American president has a more difficult time than a British prime minister in tackling smoking, because of the huge vested interests. It is a continuing battle. Ranged against the government's half-hearted commitment to combat smoking is the combined might of the multi-million pound tobacco industry – and as we have seen, that is a force to be reckoned with.

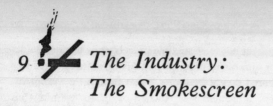

9   *The Industry: The Smokescreen*

From the first moment that cigarettes were linked with illness and especially lung cancer the cigarette manufacturers realized that were they ever to admit that the product they were promoting and selling at huge profit was dangerous, they would open the door to successful product-liability suits. From that moment their stock answer whenever questioned about the ill-effects of smoking has always been that the link between cigarettes and ill health is unproven. They often add that no one has ever been able to show exactly what is the causal mechanism. This is just a ruse to persuade the gullible that you need to know the exact mechanism to explain *how* something is dangerous before you can say that it *is* dangerous. This is illogical. You do not need to know *how* antibiotics work, for instance, to realize that they do. Nevertheless, the cigarette manufacturers believed that by pursuing this line of argument they would give comfort to smokers and defer their realization of the dangers they were running.

The 'controversy' over cigarettes is not a real controversy at all, but is manufactured by the industry to buy time and confuse smokers. For example, following the publication of the surgeon general's report in America in 1979 to mark the fifteenth anniversary of his first report, Philip Morris, the makers of Marlboro, said that in those fifteen years millions of dollars had been spent on research.

Although much of the research was concentrated on finding evidence that smoking causes disease, no conclusive medical or clinical proof has been discovered ... the tobacco industry continues to maintain the controversy can be resolved only by medical and scientific knowledge.

This last comment is designed to imply that the industry is as much concerned as anybody else to find out the truth. In fact they are concerned to do just the opposite. They have consistently denied the truth. It is hard to know what sort of proof the industry would accept.

The evidence that has accumulated satisfies practically 100 per cent of scientists worthy of the name and most of those who are not.

It could perhaps be argued that the only total proof would come from a study in which several thousand young men and women were chosen, half of them made to smoke for thirty years and half of them kept off cigarettes. You would have to ensure that they lived practically identical life styles, lived in the same place, ate the same food and exposed themselves to the same amount of environmental pollution. If more of the smokers died of lung cancer and other alleged smoking-related illnesses than the control group, then there is your proof. Such an experiment is of course impossible. Anyway, judging by the reaction of the tobacco companies to the evidence already accumulated, they would no doubt find some way of denying the evidence – perhaps by saying the two groups were not strictly comparable.

The initial reports on health and smoking in the early 1960s led to a significant drop in the sale of cigarettes immediately after their publication, but further reports had less of an impact on sales. One manufacturer believed the reason was because 'so many things have been linked to cancer that people are getting sceptical'.

Nearly twenty years after the Royal College of Physicians' first report on smoking and illness the director of research for British American Tobacco (1981 profit from tobacco £469 million), Dr Lionel Blackman (a scientist, not a medical doctor), still felt able to say that 'despite a never-ending stream of research on the possible health hazards of smoking, there is no proof of a cause-and-effect relationship between cigarette smoking and various alleged smoking diseases'.[22]

Another stock answer made by the tobacco companies when they are challenged about the health aspects of smoking is 'we are not doctors, we are not qualified to make judgements'. Yet in 1982, the trade magazine, *Tobacco*, apparently felt that it was sufficiently well qualified to pass judgement on what might happen medically to smokers who did give up. Smoking was a necessity, it said in December of that year. If smokers were forced to give up they would turn to other drugs. 'Alternatively, their withdrawal symptoms are likely to develop into personality changes which will send the divorce rate soaring, make husband-beating commonplace and fill doctors' waiting rooms with stress-related ailments.'

As the pressure built up in the early eighties, the tobacco industry formed a new group similar to its official umbrella organization, the Tobacco Advisory Council. The new group, Tobacco Alliance, was described as the communications network for the tobacco family and its allies. It was designed to provide its supporters, including employees of tobacco companies, with 'facts' and arguments 'in case they want to write to their MPs or the newspapers, or simply want to be well informed in dealing with other people's prejudices'.

With the declining sales in the late 1970s and 1980s there came a fall in employment in the tobacco industry. Between 1974 and 1983 the industry cut 14,000 jobs. There were suggestions that the total number of jobs lost was probably several times this figure if account were taken of the reduction in business for packers, distributors, retailers and so on.

Apart from the health aspects of tobacco, the industry is very concerned about the pressures building up against promotion and advertising. After the 1983 election the magazine *Tobacco*, which had so recently dispensed medical advice about the dangers of giving up smoking, urged all its readers to write to their MPs, pointing out that it was misrepresenting the case to claim, as some had done, that advertising had any influence on non-smokers. It said that every new MP would already have been, as it put it, 'assailed by the barrage of strange statistics, and the emotional and irrational arguments of the anti-smoking lobby'.

At the 1983 annual general meeting of British American Tobacco the board of directors was asked by a representative of ASH if it would give shareholders a summary of the evidence of the damage to health caused by smoking. (ASH holds one share in each of the tobacco companies so that it can have access to their company reports and annual shareholders' meetings.) The chairman of BAT, Patrick Sheehy, refused, once again falling back on an increasingly thin excuse: 'although a vast sum of money has been spent on research into the question of smoking and health, the issue is still a matter of controversy'.

At the same meeting he revealed yet more evidence of the way one arm of government is apparently opposed to smoking while another does its best to encourage the manufacture of cigarettes. He pointed out that by the autumn of 1983 the company had received over £3 million in government Regional Development Grants for its new leaf-processing plant in Corby, Northants.

The continued denial by the tobacco companies of the role of smoking in causing ill health was raised in the fourth report of the Royal College of Physicians in November 1983. The report pointed out that no tobacco company had yet accepted publicly that tobacco was harmful to health, and it cited examples of the way company officials coped with the accusations. It quoted the then chairman of Rothmans International, Sir David Nicholson, who said, speaking as a member of the European Parliament, 'There is no medical evidence to prove that a few cigarettes – say ten to fifteen a day – are bad for you.'[23] A publication produced by the Philip Morris company entitled *What About Smoking and Health?* started by saying, 'Has it been established that smoking causes cancer and other diseases? ... No ...' British American Tobacco stated in a publication produced for its employees, 'although there is a statistical association between smoking and certain kinds of ill health, it has not been proven that these illnesses are actually caused by smoking'. The Royal College of Physicians report comments,

While such an interpretation of the evidence will not deceive a well-informed public, the tragedy of developing countries is that the public there is not well informed about the dangers of smoking. When short-term economic benefits are also seen to accrue from tobacco, denials of the evidence will often meet with a sympathetic ear.

Yet once again, the RCP's strictures fell on deaf ears. The trade journal *Tobacco*, commenting on the report in January 1984, accused it of 'trotting out the usual unverifiable statistics on smoking-related premature deaths'. Another article in the same publication criticized the RCP report thus:

They are so perverse that we must use a phrase that we have used before. This is a clear case of 'don't confuse us with the facts, we have made up our minds'. But who are 'they'? Is the Royal College of Physicians really speaking for its large body of hospital staff and family physician members? Most of those we meet seem to be, in the main, tolerant people open to discussion and fully understanding that smoking and health is a subject about which too little is known for sweeping generalizations and half-cock statistical claims.

The industry frequently accuses the medical profession of making sweeping generalizations based on 'statistics', used here in the perjorative sense, yet itself extrapolates wildly from certain scientific statements, using them to justify almost anything. For example, when the Froggat Committee, an independent committee on smoking, said in one of its reports in 1984 that nicotine itself had not been shown to harm the cardiovascular system in healthy people, the magazine *Tobacco* used this one phrase to justify a plea that a smoking ban in hospitals should be resisted. The magazine claimed that 'not only patients but hospital staff as well find relief from stress in the nicotine which the independent scientific committee has so significantly failed to condemn'. The magazine clearly failed to realize that nicotine was only one of some 3,000 chemicals present in tobacco smoke.

There was one occasion, however, when the tobacco industry, or at least an organization close to it, let its armour slip, revealing what everyone recognizes and the industry must know in its heart. Stephen Eyres, director of FOREST – the 'freedom' organization set up in 1979 to campaign on behalf of smokers – revealed that he at least did accept that smoking caused premature death. At a meeting at which he addressed a sub-committee of the Tory think-tank on the subject of deregulating tobacco, he was quoted as pointing out what he presumably saw as an advantage of this – that it would reduce the overall cost of the Health Service. One can hardly think of a more cynical comment to come from the spokesman of an organization supported so whole-heartedly by the tobacco industry, although it was said at the time to be a joke. He also pointed out that the taxes paid by smokers, over £4,000 million, far outweighed the costs to the health service of smoking (£155–300 million).

By 1984 the medical pressure had obviously become so irritating to the tobacco companies that one of them, R. J. Reynolds, decided to finance a $20 million advertising campaign intended to discredit and challenge the medical evidence about smoking. The company placed full-page advertisements arguing the case for smoking in national magazines and metropolitan newspapers in America. One read, 'Over the years you have heard so many negative reports about smoking and health and so little to challenge these reports that you may assume that the case against smoking is closed. This is far from the truth.' The advertisements argued that the evidence of a link between smoking and various diseases was statistical and that no causal connection could be shown. They said that there was 'considerable evidence to contradict the common assumption that smoking is bad for you'. Health organizations joined forces to condemn the advertisements as the most misleading and irresponsible advertising campaigns in memory.

In Britain in 1984 the Consumers Association took the Tobacco Advisory Council to task for the way in which it misleadingly and selectively quoted the results of a survey it had carried out into people's opinions about smoking. For example, in one of its advertisements the Tobacco Advisory Council said, 'Did you know that over nine out of ten smokers agreed "people should be free to choose whether they smoke or not"?' But *Which?* magazine, published by the Consumers' Association, quoted other results from the survey, which showed its overall message in a very different light. For example, almost everyone agreed that 'there should be no smoking in food shops', and nine out of ten agreed that there should be no-smoking areas in cinemas. The Consumers' Association commented, 'It's not quite the same thing is it?'

The tobacco industry will go to enormous lengths to suppress what it sees as threats to its well being. On one occasion in 1984 in Australia it went that bit too far and received a warning from the speaker of the Legislative Assembly in New South Wales. The incident arose over the Thames Television film *Death in the West*. This film had been made in 1976 and showed that the healthy cowboy riding the range with a Marlboro cigarette dangling from his lips was a myth. Thames Television had found and interviewed cowboys who had smoked much of their lives, and who were dying of cancer. Philip Morris had been so appalled by the film that it had taken out an injunction in London preventing Thames Television from selling the film or showing it again. Pirated copies of the film were made and over the years it has received a wide television showing all over the world. Philip Morris was apparently powerless to prevent this, but when an Australian MP, Mr Ernie Page, planned to screen the film in the parliamentary theatre, the company threatened to bring an injunction against him. The speaker informed solicitors acting for the company that their actions constituted a gross breach of privilege.

The tobacco industry has a habit of criticizing others for using tactics it has no qualms about using itself. For example, in 1985 the organization FOREST attacked the professionalism with which Britain's annual No-Smoking Day is organized. Professionalism in persuading people to buy cigarettes, as demonstrated by the cute way the tobacco industry gets round voluntary agreements and legislation banning television advertising is one thing, but apparently when anti-smoking organizations start getting professional that is another. No-Smoking Day in 1985 was 20 March. FOREST described it as 'the most lavish, professional, intensive and costly campaign ever against Britain's seventeen million smokers'. Its newspaper said, 'the organized propagandists have taken over ... Weeks of nagging and nannying, hectoring and lecturing, coercing and cajoling lie ahead.' The irony was apparently lost on the writers of that article.

In the same issue FOREST attacked the money the government had given to ASH, once again conveniently neglecting to compare the grant of £136,000 with the multi-million pound advertising budgets of the tobacco industry. The article's particular point was that the grant had been increased at a rate higher than the rate of inflation. It said that MPs were concerned about this but gave only limited evidence to this effect.

This issue of the newspaper also carried a story claiming that research in Minnesota purported to show that smokers were more productive than non-smokers. The study of fifty-five managers seemed to show that they were '3 per cent more effective at making use of their time than non-smokers' – presumably because they knew that they did not have as much time left to them to be productive in as non-smokers!

The tobacco industry in Britain spends well over £100 million a year on advertising and promotion, including sponsorship of sport and the arts. Compared with this colossal sum, the amount of money spent on persuading people not to smoke is paltry. In 1983 ASH received a grant of £135,000. The Health Education Council had a grant of only £8.5 million for all its activities and the Scottish Health Education Group £2 million. In 1981 nearly a quarter of all poster advertising was for cigarettes. In America the figures are even more startling. There the tobacco industry spent no less than $2.7 billion on advertising in 1983, nearly 25 per cent up on the previous year, in an attempt to counteract a fall in the sale of cigarettes. Advertising in newspapers and magazines alone cost $750 million – more than is spent to advertise any other product including cars.

The most famous cigarette advertisement of all – the Marlboro cowboy – was conceived in 1954 in America. The chairman of Philip Morris, George Weissman, said at the time that the cowboy was chosen as an advertising symbol 'because he is close to the earth'. By 1980 more than 100 billion Marlboro cigarettes were being sold in America each year and seventy billion in the rest of the world. In Britain advertising started in earnest in 1955 when tobacco became more plentiful after the war.

The first report of the Royal College of Physicians in 1962 drew attention to the fact that between 1955 and 1960 expenditure on cigarette advertising had tripled, and while no advertisement specifically encouraged heavier smoking, the report noted that there had been a subtle change in the advertising. It was increasingly aimed at young people and cigarettes were being given a romantic setting. A month after the Royal College of Physicians report was published the tobacco industry agreed to a voluntary code of practice on advertising which excluded advertisements that over-emphasized the pleasure of smoking, contained figures whom the young might consider heroes, or appealed to manliness, romance and social success.

In Britain efforts to get the tobacco companies to restrict television advertising to periods after nine o'clock failed when the companies refused to co-operate. Cigarette advertisements on television were finally banned in 1965. Five years later America followed suit.

However, many anti-smoking organizations have been urging a total ban on all advertising – in the media, on posters and on bill-boards. It is something the tobacco companies have been fighting hard. Their argument has always been that advertising does not encourage people to smoke but merely influences people's choice of brands. The anti-smoking groups claim that advertisements have a particular influence on the young and that this is the group the tobacco companies want to influence, because once young people are hooked, the chances are they will continue to smoke, ensuring a profitable future for the tobacco companies.

Politicians have always been reluctant to institute any sort of ban on advertising, preferring to accept the industry's word that this would not reduce overall consumption. However, in 1975 Dr David Owen, then minister of health, changed this attitude by saying, 'there is good evidence that cigarette advertising increases cigarette smoking'. Surveys have shown that a majority of people would favour a restriction or a ban on advertising cigarettes. One of the most important effects of a ban might be to finally persuade smokers that smoking is bad for you – a survey in 1983 showed that 44 per cent of smokers agreed that 'smoking cannot be really dangerous or the government would ban cigarette advertising'. This gives added impetus to the British Medical Association's claims that so long as the government avoids any serious restrictions on tobacco promotion, 'its commitment to reducing smoking remains empty rhetoric'.

Apart from their claim that advertising only encourages people to change brands, not to take up smoking or smoke more, the tobacco industry uses several other arguments to justify its policy of advertising cigarettes. First, it maintains that so long as cigarettes are legal products it should be legal to advertise them. Second, advertising is aimed at adults and not children, and third, advertisements provide information for smokers, encouraging their conversion to lower-tar brands.

In fact, the true reason why companies continue to advertise is to promote smoking. In a speech at the Wholesale Tobacco Trade Annual Dinner Dance the managing director of Carreras Rothman, K. S. Blair, commented on widely advertised cuts in the price of cigarettes after the 1976 budget, saying, 'the aim to keep people smoking has been achieved'. Several advertising executives have dismissed the tobacco industry's claims that it only advertises to increase market share, and not to encourage people to smoke. One claimed that the idea was 'so preposterous it is insulting'. Another claimed that creating positive climates of social acceptability for smokers would encourage new smokers and that this is more important to the tobacco companies than simply increasing market share.

A recent *British Medical Journal* report pointed out that advertising undermines government health policies, contradicts advice to children from parents and teachers, and discourages people from believing that smoking is dangerous to health. All the major international health, cancer and heart-disease agencies, medical colleges and consumer organizations, notably the World Health Organization and the World Health Assembly, have agreed that all forms of tobacco promotion should be banned.

In 1982 forty-seven countries had laws or voluntary agreements restricting certain kinds of tobacco advertising. Of these, twenty-one have banned tobacco advertising completely including Finland, Iceland, Italy, Norway, Senegal, Singapore, Somalia, Sudan and Yugoslavia.

In 1984 the junior health minister, John Patten, gave another example of how immune the government seems to be to persuasion by medical experts, and of how it accepts instead the advice of the tobacco industry. He told Parliament that there was no clear evidence that a ban on advertising would reduce the incidence of smoking. He claimed that in countries such as Norway, where there is an advertising ban, the decline in smoking had been much less than in Britain over the same period. What the anti-smoking lobby claim is that in Norway the ban on advertising had produced a dramatic fall in the number of children smoking, and also that during this period there had been big increases in taxes on cigarettes in Britain, which had cut sales. The 1983 Royal College of Physicians report said, 'if an advertising ban affected only the uptake of smoking by children the ultimate benefit to mankind would be enormous, and the importance of introducing legislation to enact such a ban cannot be over-emphasized'.

There have been a number of voluntary agreements between the government and the cigarette companies over advertising and promotion. In 1977 the then social services secretary, David (now Lord) Ennals, announced a tightening-up of the code governing advertising. The existing code already forbade advertisements which suggested that cigarette smoking implied social or business success, or which depicted contemporary figures admired by young people. The new code went a good deal further. It banned advertisements which implied that one cigarette was safer or more healthy than any other, or in which smoking appeared to enhance female charm and it stopped the depiction of smokers as participants or spectators at sporting events.

In 1980 a further agreement was announced under which there would be a 30 per cent reduction in poster advertising and no cigarette posters would be placed near schools or playgrounds. There would be new and more varied warnings on cigarette packets and posters, restrictions on cigarette promotions aimed at young people and on promotional offers generally, and there would be an intensified programme to reduce the tar yields of cigarettes. The industry agreed to take steps to discourage manufacturers of non-tobacco products from including tobacco brand names or designs on goods with a special appeal for young people. From the time of its announcement the agreement had one year and eight months to run – although the industry fought long and hard for a four-year agreement.

A new agreement was negotiated in October 1982 with the new minister of health, Kenneth Clarke, whose commitment against smoking appeared to many people to be much less convincing than that of some of his predecessors. The agreement was to last for three and a half years. It meant more space for warnings on cigarette packets, a further progressive reduction on poster and cinema advertising and a reduction in the tar ceiling above which a cigarette brand was not allowed to be advertised.

However, the main part of Mr Clarke's announcement was heavily criticized. It concerned the setting up of the so-called Health Promotion Research Trust with £11 million of tobacco-industry money, to conduct a 'balanced' programme of research into ways of encouraging people, especially young people, to adopt a more responsible attitude to promoting and maintaining their own health. Mr Clarke described the trust as an important new development and said it would provide 'a valuable supplement to the health-research effort at a time when resources are scarce'. It was a triumph for the tobacco companies in terms of public-relations: it made the industry appear philanthropic, yet the trust was specifically excluded from doing any studies designed 'directly or indirectly to examine the use and effects of tobacco products'. Anti-smoking organizations called it 'blood money'. Dr Keith Ball, the vice-president of ASH, said, 'it is beyond belief that the tobacco industry has the sheer effrontery to claim an interest in health promotion when it excludes from research the major avoidable cause of ill health in Britian today'. A letter in the *Lancet* compared it with the Mafia sponsoring research into law and order but ruling out organized crime.

Some time after the trust was set up two of its original trustees, Dr Jonathan Miller and Professor Eva Alberman, resigned when they recognized the significance of where the money was coming from. In December 1985 the leading article in the *British Medical Journal* made a blistering attack on the trust. It set out three reasons why researchers should not accept grants from the trust: it buys the tobacco industry respectability; money from the trust might buy off an influential and articulate opponent of the industry; and this 'dirty' money could influence research. At least one distinguished researcher, Professor Hilary Rose of Bradford University, sent back £30,000 of trust money she had been granted to carry out research into the alcohol problems of women. However, many researchers still accept money from it and, as the *BMJ* pointed out, two doctors remain on the trust: its chairman, Sir John Butterfield, and Professor Arthur Buller.

Despite the agreements on advertising, experience shows that whatever the advertising code says, the industry makes every effort to circumvent it once the agreement is signed. For example, the code prohibits the cigarette companies from investing their advertisements with any glamour, yet when Carreras Rothman launched a £5 million press-and-poster campaign for Peter Stuyvesant luxury length cigarettes, a spokesman for the advertisers was quoted in *Marketing* magazine as saying, 'We are injecting style, internationalism and quality'. The advertisements highlight the cigarette's extra length, but as the spokesman explained, 'this emphasis on length isn't meant to have any erotic symbolism – it merely reflects the prime position of the pack'.

Even restricting the type and content of the advertisements can have a measurable effect on sales. In 1979, for example, Sweden introduced regulations which restricted the size of advertisements in newspapers and magazines and only permitted the advertisement to depict the cigarette packet against a plain background. In the following year the number of smokers fell by 6 per cent. The apparent decline among children was more encouraging. In Finland cigarette advertising was banned in March 1978, as were other forms of promotion, such as using non-tobacco goods like holidays or sports-wear and clothing to promote a brand name or image. Again, statistics show that there was a steady decline in smoking: in 1973 19 per cent of fourteen-year-olds were daily smokers; by 1979 the number had dropped by more than half, to 8 per cent.

Laws banning advertising have not always been implemented as firmly as intended. In Italy, for example, tobacco advertising has been outlawed for the past sixteen years but the fine for breaking the law was so small that many companies made allowances for it in their budgets. In 1983 fines were increased to between £2,000 and £20,000, the average being about £4,000. As a result advertising agencies, publications and television channels paid out over £1.5 million in fines that year for 'advertisements' where cigarette packets had been slipped into advertisements for other products such as holidays.

Because of the considerable decline in sales in the early 1980s tobacco companies in America became really worried and decided to pull out all the stops to restore their position in the market. Their advertising budget soared. Once again they tried to associate their products with healthy outdoor activities like sport. One advertisement featured the slogan 'Alive with pleasure' and was illustrated by a young man and woman involved in many outdoor activities. Virginia Slims, a Philip Morris product aimed at women, featured the slogan 'You've come a long way, baby'.

From an early stage tobacco companies realized the potential in the women's market. Cigarettes designed especially for women have become more popular. In 1983 an article in the industry's trade journal

Tobacco pointed out the value of the woman's market, stressing that far fewer women were giving up smoking than men and that those who did smoke were either smoking more cigarettes or smoking more tobacco as they switched from small economy brands to extra-longs. Women are believed to buy more than half the extra-long cigarettes. Women are much more financially independent than they used to be, and the article pointed out that since the 1950s, during the long period of publicity about the ill effects of smoking, women's cigarette-consumption in Britain and other Western countries actually increased. One reason could well be the extensive advertising of cigarettes in women's magazines. More than half the women in Britain read a women's magazine and the tobacco industry has not been slow to exploit this. Between 1977 and 1982 tobacco companies increased their spending on advertisements in women's magazines by 50 per cent, to £4.5 million. By 1984 the tobacco companies were spending nearly £7 million. Women traditionally regard women's magazines as a reliable source of information and advice, especially about personal matters like health. The magazines' dependence on advertising means that many are reluctant to carry articles about the dangers of smoking – the one subject where they could have a marked impact. In 1985 a British Medical Association survey showed that only a third of the magazines they investigated refused cigarette advertising, and those were mostly magazines aimed at teenagers. However, many of the magazines which do accept cigarette advertisements have a high proportion of young readers. When asked to justify why *Woman's Realm* accepts cigarette advertisements, the editor replied, 'Yes, I do accept advertising for products known to be hazardous to health, not just cigarettes but also alcohol, butter, cream and all dairy products.'

In their efforts to fight a ban on advertising the tobacco companies sometimes play on people's fear of 'big brother' by asking, if there is a ban on cigarette advertising, where will it stop? They suggest that it could be on other dangerous products like cars, cycles, alcohol, sugar and so on. They fail to point out, of course, that all these other products are safe when used properly and barring accidents. Tobacco is the only advertised product which is hazardous when used as intended.

Whatever restrictions are placed on the advertising policies of

tobacco companies, they will always find a way of exploiting loopholes.
Even if they abide by the letter of an agreement they certainly do not
abide by its spirit. For example, the code governing the advertising
of cigarettes states that 'no advertisement should appear in any
publication directed wholly or mainly at young people'. The loophole
through which the advertisers crawl is the fact that there is no
definition of what is meant by young people. The United Nations
designates twenty-five as the upper limit of youth. By this definition
the advertising code is being widely broken. However, following
complaints, the Advertising Standards Association announced that
the United Nations definition of youth was not relevant to the code.
The association preferred to define young people as those under
eighteen.

Some of these problems – the definition of what is meant by young
people and the advertising of cigarettes in women's magazines – were
tackled in 1986 in the new agreement negotiated between the
Department of Health and the tobacco industry and announced by
the social services secretary, Norman Fowler, on 24 March. Under
the terms of the agreement the industry agreed not to advertise
cigarettes in magazines with a female readership of more than 200,000
where a third or more of the readers were aged between fifteen and
twenty-four years.

The other provisions included new health warnings for cigarette
packets and advertisements, replacing the single health warning from
HM Government. The new warnings are ascribed to the Health
Department's chief medical officers. Cigarette packets will now bear
one of six possible warnings: 'Smoking can cause fatal diseases',
'Smoking can cause heart diseases', 'Smoking when pregnant can
injure your baby and cause premature birth', 'Stopping smoking
reduces the risk of serious diseases', 'Smoking can cause lung cancer,
bronchitis and other chest diseases', and 'More than 30,000 people
die each year from lung cancer'. The space devoted to the health
warning and tar ratings on posters and press advertisements is to be
increased from 15 per cent to 17.5 per cent.

Among the other provisions in the agreement were a ban on cinema
advertising, a freeze on spending on poster advertising, new rules
preventing cigarette posters being put up near schools, no cigarette-
brand advertising or logos on 'giveaways' to children at events

sponsored by tobacco companies such as roadshows and airshows, and no advertising for cigarettes yielding 18 mg tar or more.

In addition, the industry agreed to spend £1 million a year for the three and a half years of the agreement on a campaign aimed at retailers to stop the sale of cigarettes to children under sixteen. Finally, for the first time a committee was established to monitor the agreement. The committee is to be made up of industry and Department of Health experts under an independent chairman, who will report annually.

Norman Fowler described the agreement as 'a considerable advance' on the previous one, particularly because of the steps it had taken to help protect vulnerable groups such as children and young women. The anti-smoking organization, Action on Smoking and Health, described the agreement as a step in the right direction but warned that the industry would find ways of getting round it and regretted that it did nothing to prevent the tobacco industry promoting cigarettes through travel holidays and leisure wear. The British Medical Association was also wary of it, claiming that it did little more than paper over the cracks in the previous highly unsatisfactory agreement.

After cigarette advertising was banned from British television screens in 1965 the companies devised alternative promotional schemes, notably the coupon scheme. Each cigarette packet contained coupons which the smoker saved until he had enough for a 'free gift'. By 1966 the tobacco industry was spending over £20 million a year on cigarette-coupon schemes, which quite blatantly encouraged people to smoke more. From 1965 to 1966 cigarette sales increased by six billion. In 1973, when Value Added Tax was introduced, coupon schemes became taxable and commercially unattractive. When tax increases began to bite in 1978 coupons virtually died a death, but companies had begun to explore other ways of promoting their products, from the sponsorship of sports and other events to promoting a range of other goods carrying the cigarette brand-name, logo or colours.

In May 1979 at a five-day conference held in Germany executives of BAT discussed the increasing restrictions they were facing. They even contemplated the possibility of beaming television advertisements by satellite into countries where they were banned. They also discussed the possibility of attaching the cigarette brand-name, logo and colours to other non-tobacco products, which they termed back-door advertising.

Two months later BAT Cigaretten-Fabriken licensed an Italian fashion marketing group, Kim Modo of Milan, to use the logo and colours of Kim, one of its best-selling brands aimed at women. Kim cigarettes were launched in Britain in the summer of 1982, just before the Wimbledon tennis championships, where several of the players were to wear sports clothes emblazoned with the 'Kim' logo. Although this breached the sponsorship agreement, BAT denied the events were connected or that it had anything to do with the agreement between the tennis stars and the Italian fashion company. It did make an apology to the sports minister, Neil Macfarlane, but the following year a row again broke out at Wimbledon when Martina Navratilova opened the championship wearing a tennis dress that was almost identical. It bore the symbol and colours of Kim cigarettes but the word 'Kim' had been replaced by the word 'Topline'. ASH protested, saying that even though the name was no longer in evidence, the colour and style of the outfit were unmistakeably connected with the current advertising for a cigarette brand and betrayed the spirit of the voluntary agreement. The matter was raised in Parliament by Laurie Pavitt, MP, who said that the tobacco industry had run rings around the government and that the voluntary agreement was not worth the paper it was written on. By the end of the championship Miss Navratilova was wearing a white dress.

If BAT began the trend of exploiting fashion as a way of promoting cigarettes, Peter Stuyvesant was the first company to see the possibility of brand promotion through the travel trade. Soon Gallaher and Philip Morris followed suit. In 1983 the British Medical Association attacked tobacco companies for using 'sly' methods of promoting cigarettes. Philip Morris, for example, had started up Marlboro Adventure Holidays and was advertising them on television. A spokesman for Gallaher justified their particular holiday promotion by saying that 'names like Silk Cut and Benson and Hedges are known and recognized for their quality and reliability. We consider it is entirely reasonable for us to build independent new businesses on those names.'

To show the cynical lengths to which tobacco companies go an advertisement by the BAT group in West Germany would be hard to beat. In a campaign organized in conjunction with a local supermarket a poster depicted an open packet of cigarettes together with a bunch of grapes, cheese, nuts and wine, with the slogan 'good things belong together'.

In 1983 Benson and Hedges bought advertisements in four daily newspapers in Australia during a royal tour. The papers carried large colour pictures of the Prince and Princess of Wales together with Prince William on a page adjacent to a large colour advertisement for Benson and Hedges. It looked as though the royal tour were being sponsored by Benson and Hedges. It had not escaped the advertisers' notice that children would be keeping pictures of the royal couple; indeed the photographs were being pinned up in classrooms throughout the country. One doctor claimed it meant that Benson and Hedges had advertisements for their products in schools all over Australia.

Cigarette companies will apparently stop at nothing to try to seem as respectable as possible while peddling their unhealthy products. During a televised debate in Hong Kong, for example, the research director of the Advertising Association, Mr Mike Waterson, claimed that there was no real evidence to show that cigarette advertising encouraged people to smoke. In support of this statement he said, 'Martin Plant of the Royal Edinburgh Hospital, one of the very few doctors who has actually taken the trouble to look at the evidence in this area as opposed to making claims, summarized the evidence in a recent book. He said that the effects of advertising, if not non-existent, were at best trivial.' But Martin Plant protested to both the Advertising Association and the television station. His work, he said, related to the advertising of alcohol not tobacco; to call him a doctor in this context was misleading, as people would assume he was a medical doctor whereas he was a sociologist. In any case, he disapproved of smoking: he said the damage to health from cigarette smoking was massive and appalling and he 'did not sympathize in any way with either the concealment of this fact or the promotion of this form of lethal behaviour'.

Tobacco companies have tried to exploit loopholes in the voluntary agreements by advertising cigarettes without putting a health warning on the advertisement. For example, for a while in 1984 gold-painted taxis were driving around London with the words 'Benson and Hedges' on their sides but without any health warning. Junior Health Minister Mr John Patten said that he had been informed that the taxis 'were intended to publicize the name of the company which had a range of trading activities including the manufacture of cigarettes and other tobacco products'. The company was eventually told that the government regarded the taxis as a direct advertisement for Benson and Hedges cigarettes, whereupon it decided to change the door panels to overt advertisements for the cigarette brand and include a health warning.

The cigarette companies have developed a new form of advertisement which they call 'advertorials' – a cross between an advertisement and editorial copy. The August 1985 issue of *Options* magazine, for example, had a four-page promotion, each page carrying the logo of Raffles cigarettes. The magazine admitted that the manufacturers had paid in part for the promotion. It claimed that because it was not an advertisement it did not have to carry a government health warning and it did not have to abide by the government's voluntary agreement with the tobacco industry. In this way the magazine, which has a readership of 845,000 of which 40 per cent are under twenty-five, became a powerful advertising tool of the industry. Raffles admitted they had been involved in several other promotions during the year.

As the government places more restrictions on what is allowed by way of advertising, the companies will always find ways of circumventing the agreements. Rothmans, for example, has pointed to the potential of marketing point-of-sale displays more appealingly: improving the 'dramatic effect' of shelving, for example, by using fibre optics, holograms and chip technology. It also believes staff might be used more creatively, by wearing branded overalls, for example.

The most effective method of influencing the public to buy tobacco products has proved to be sponsorship both of sport and the arts. Indeed, so successful has it been that some would say it is far more cost-effective than straightforward advertising. In the 1970s overall sponsorship of sports and the arts grew at about 20 per cent a year. The £15 million spent in 1973 had risen to £50 million by 1981, 90 per cent of which was devoted to sports sponsorship. Tobacco companies were by far the biggest sponsors.

In 1977 Social Services Secretary David Ennals made some harsh comments about the sponsorship of sports by tobacco companies. 'It seems to me,' he said, 'that this practice is not merely an evasion of the spirit of the ban on television advertising, but that it is grotesque for outdoor sports to be so closely associated with habits that are notoriously dangerous to health.'

That year an agreement was negotiated between the tobacco industry and the Department of the Environment, bringing sports sponsorship under some sort of control. The agreement was renegotiated in 1982 and again in 1985. Under the 1977 agreement the companies said they would keep their spending in real terms within the levels reached in 1976 and they also agreed not to display their brand names at televised events or on competitors and their equipment.

By 1981 sports sponsorship was effectively giving the tobacco companies 247 hours of television time a year through nationwide coverage of sports sponsored by them. Imperial, the makers of Embassy and John Player, had 116 hours of screen time. Gallaher received fifty-five hours for Benson and Hedges, and British American Tobacco forty-five hours for State Express. That year the BBC carried seventy-two hours of Embassy snooker, thirty-six hours of State Express snooker, thirty-three hours of John Player cricket, twenty hours of Benson and Hedges cricket, twelve hours of Benson and Hedges tennis, twelve hours of Benson and Hedges snooker, eleven hours of Benson and Hedges golf, eleven hours of Embassy darts and nine hours of State Express golf.

In 1983 eight of the top twenty-three televised sporting events were sponsored by tobacco companies and received over 233 hours of television coverage. In 1984 television coverage of fourteen sports events sponsored by tobacco companies totalled 323 hours. Yet in one way the sponsorship has been too successful for the tobacco companies' own good. *Marketing* magazine has pointed out that if tobacco companies were banned from sponsoring sporting events, so prominent have the events become in the public mind that their organizers would not have to wait very long for substitute sponsors to step in.

Apart from coverage on television, sponsored events also receive wide publicity in newspapers. In one three-week period in December 1982, for example, no fewer than fifteen sports events sponsored by tobacco companies received press coverage. They included the Embassy World Professional Darts Championship, bowls, cricket, rugby, tennis, snooker, bobsleigh, motor sports of various kinds, sailing and horse racing.

The absurdity of enforcing a ban on straightforward advertising of cigarettes while coverage of sponsored sports gives the tobacco companies such massive publicity drove the medical authorities to protest. In 1981, as negotiations on a new agreement began, the presidents of the eight Royal Colleges wrote to Neil MacFarlane, the new sports minister, saying they were concerned that sponsorship by tobacco interests would lead young people to associate smoking with participation in healthy sports. But their protests had little effect. In 1982 a new sponsorship agreement lasting three years was signed.

The 1982 agreement covered various aspects of sports sponsorship. For example, it was agreed that the expenditure on sponsorship should not exceed the 1976 level, with allowances made for inflation, and that media, advertising and promotional material had to be a reasonable proportion of the total amount spent on sponsoring that event. The companies were obliged to notify the Department of the Environment of any changes in their future plans; all the advertising signs at sponsored events and promotional signs had to carry health warnings; the number, siting and size of signs at televised sporting events were restricted; at televised events no participant or piece of equipment was to carry house names, brand names of symbols. There were controls on which sports could be sponsored – none where the majority of participants were under eighteen – and the companies were to continue to sponsor non-televised events and activities of minor or amateur interest. However, the tobacco companies were to be allowed to call an event after a brand name rather than just the house or company name.

In his book *The Smoke Ring* Peter Taylor quotes a spokesman at the Department of the Environment who justified the agreement by saying, 'sport needs all the money it can get, smoking tobacco is a perfectly legal activity, sport is a perfectly legal activity, so there is nothing illegal or undesirable in one legal activity sponsoring another'. It is an argument many disagree with, including at least one former social services secretary (David Ennals).

In November 1983 the Central Council for Physical Recreation commissioned a report under the chairmanship of the former sports minister, Mr Denis Howell, to look at the various ethical considerations surrounding sports sponsorship. Not surprisingly, the report was sympathetic to sponsorship of sport by tobacco interests. It stressed that it thought sponsorship by the tobacco industry should be regulated by voluntary agreement and added, 'where a pursuit is lawful and especially when the government itself derives substantial income from such pursuits there can be no objection in principle to the sponsorship of sport from any sources. The freedom of sport and sports people to determine these questions for themselves must be safeguarded.'

Following the Howell report on sports sponsorship the Sports Council set up a working party to consider its recommendations. One of the matters for discussion was the rule governing the use of product names and the number of times a sponsor's name might be mentioned during the course of a programme. Current regulations can sometimes be so contradictory. For example, new sponsors can use company names but usually not product names, although tobacco manufacturers are able to name events after their brands.

In 1984 the third agreement was negotiated. Once again this restricted expenditure to the 1976 level allowing for inflation; it stipulated that the government health warning should appear on the advertisements for the sponsored events and on promotional signs at these events; it called on the companies to restrict expenditure on media advertising and promotional activities to a reasonable proportion of total sponsorship expenditure; it imposed specific limitations on the amount of promotional material at televised events, placed controls on what sort of sports could be sponsored and called on companies not to sponsor activities in which the majority of participants were under the age of eighteen.

The tobacco companies have been adept at sidestepping the agreements on occasions and, like the agreements on advertising, exploiting gaps. There are many instances where the ethics of the tobacco companies have been dubious to say the least. One illustration was provided in 1983, when George Faulkes, MP, pointed out that an event known as 'Snow Fun Week' at Glenshee, sponsored by Peter Stuyvesant and billed as 'skiing and fun for the family', breached the sponsorship agreement because many of the events were open to children as well as adults and there had even been a special children's day. There had been extensive cigarette promotion during the week.

Just occasionally the tobacco industry would find their apparent philanthropy backfiring on them. At one tennis match – the 1983 Benson and Hedges Tennis Championships at Wembley – the two players, John McEnroe and Steve Denton, complained about the spectators smoking. Denton claimed it was like playing in a London fog. Calm returned when the extractor fans were turned on, but the publicity this little fracas attracted must have cancelled out any benefit the company might have hoped for.

Even sports that at one time refused sponsorship from tobacco companies found themselves drawn into the net by enthusiastic marketing executives. Professional basketball, for example, had initially refused tobacco sponsorship but when it found it could not obtain support from anywhere else, it changed its mind. A director of the basketball marketing company was quoted as saying, 'a survey has shown that 60 per cent of our supporters are between the ages of eighteen and twenty-five, which makes it an ideal market for tobacco and drinks companies'.

If there were any doubt as to the real reason why tobacco companies sponsor sporting events, a paragraph in *The Times* in July 1985 gave the game away. Photographers covering the test match at Old Trafford were reminded they would be allowed to stand on the boundary only on the understanding that they did not obscure advertising hoardings from the BBC television cameras.

In December 1985 the Health Education Council launched a campaign to stop the BBC promoting cigarettes on television. In a letter to the BBC it called for an end to the widespread violation of the guidelines which restrict TV advertisements. It pointed out that in 1984 the tobacco companies received 330 hours of television coverage for the sports they sponsored, most of it on BBC programmes. It accused the BBC of making a mockery of the ban on advertising cigarettes on television. The code which governs cigarette advertising elsewhere makes it clear that cigarettes should not be associated with sport, fitness, manliness, courage, daring or heroes of the young. But because sports sponsorship is not 'proper' advertising the industry is able to associate these qualities with cigarettes. The code is meant to protect children from tobacco promotion, but research has shown that the 1984 Embassy World Professional Snooker championship was watched at some point by nearly half of all young people between the ages of seven and fifteen. The HEC is also concerned that the promotion of cigarettes began to creep on to children's programmes in 1985, when the *Late Late Breakfast Show* gave coverage to the

Marlboro aerobatic team and the Peter Stuyvesant ski display. The HEC believes these were blatant attempts by the industry to overcome the present ban on cigarette advertising.

Sponsorship goes far wider than just sporting events. It has invaded the arts in a big way and in some ways the impact is more subtle. While sponsorship of the arts does not seek to link cigarettes with a health-giving activity like sport, it does ensnare arts organizations, which might find great difficulty in getting sponsorship from other sources, particularly as the arts do not have the popular appeal of sports. The arts are a minority interest, but by sponsorship of various artistic endeavours tobacco companies seek to associate their products with respectability.

Three of London's main orchestras are sponsored by tobacco companies. Imperial tobacco puts money into the English, Welsh and Scottish National Operas, the National Theatre, the Glyndebourne Festival Opera, the London Philharmonic Orchestra, Sadlers Wells, Ballet Rambert, the John Player Portrait Awards and John Player classical records. Rothmans sponsors opera scholarships and Gallaher sponsors the Benson and Hedges Music Festival at Aldeburgh. Imperial Tobacco's former chairman and managing director, Tony Garrett, sits on the board of the Glyndebourne Arts Trust. Imperial invites dozens of MPs to be its guests for an evening at the opera, including three who went on to become ministers of health: Patrick Jenkin, David Ennals and Gerard Vaughan.

The publicity that sponsored events attract is also an important reason why the tobacco companies maintain their presence in the arts. Indeed, when there is no publicity they think again. In November 1984 Benson and Hedges decided to withdraw its sponsorship from an international operatic competition, the Gold Award singing competition, apparently because it failed to attract television coverage and there had been criticism that the event might be seen to link vocal ability and smoking.

There have been many other sponsoring ventures. The 'Marlboro Challenge', for example, in which Philip Morris selects twenty entrants to train as motor-sports drivers. A spokesman for the company justified this by saying that large organizations like Philip Morris had 'a wider role in society' to fulfil. He maintained that the Marlboro Challenge had no clear commercial purpose. The entrants are selected from the thousands of people who apply by means of some twelve million leaflets distributed through pubs, clubs and sweet shops.

Tobacco companies sponsor book publishing – especially books on sport and sports annuals. *Tobacco* magazine commented that such books are a good medium because they are relatively inexpensive compared to most advertising costs, they come out every year, and they are rarely thrown away. The books range from the *Macmillan and Silk Cut Nautical Almanac* to the *Rothmans Rugby League Year Book*. Tourist guides are another line. In 1983 Gallaher promised three years of financial aid in the name of Benson and Hedges to the British Tourist Authority to assist in the publication of the authority's guide *Stay at the Inn*.

However, the pressure against sponsorship, and particularly sports sponsorship, is building up and it can only be a matter of time before the government cracks down on it in response to the huge amount of lobbying by health organizations and others, many of whom claim considerable public support. When the British Medical Association launched its anti-smoking campaign on 16 October 1984 one under-secretary, Dr John Dawson, described the cosy voluntary agreements on sports sponsorship between successive governments and the cigarette manufacturers as 'a sick joke'.

The BMA announced that it was starting talks with the BBC and the IBA on tobacco sponsorship of televised events. Mr Peter Lawson, the general secretary of the Central Council for Physical Recreation, has said, 'No credible evidence has ever been produced to indicate that the enjoyment by the viewing public of televised events sponsored by the tobacco industry induces people to take up smoking.' Researchers at the London Polytechnic have pointed out the lack of evidence concerning the relationship between cigarette promotion and cigarette consumption is not surprising given that 'tobacco companies do not make available data on sponsorship expenditure or promotions and poster advertising expenditure to independent researchers unless the companies are granted the right to veto any research results'.

Sports bodies claim that sponsorship is valuable and they could not do the work they do without it. Those who favour a ban on sponsorship maintain that if taxation on cigarette packets were increased by 0.1p an additional £6 million would be raised – enough to pay for all the tobacco industry spends on sports and arts sponsorship.

The health lobby has won a significant battle in Canada, where the government has announced that tobacco-company sponsorship of amateur sport will be phased out. When the parliament of Western Australia began considering banning all tobacco promotion the tobacco companies tried to intimidate the sports-mad Australians by claiming that the ban would devastate their favourite pastime. The Australian Cricket Board did little to dissipate the scaremongering by claiming that Perth might lose its test match if the legislation went through. The industry also claimed that racing would be threatened, although the racing authorities denied this, saying that there would be a queue of replacement sponsors.

Not all those who benefit from taking part in fields of endeavour sponsored by tobacco companies approve of where the money is coming from. In the arts world a strong lobby has developed called 'Artists' Campaign Against Tobacco Sponsorship'. This has pledged to fight sponsorship even though it may mean less work for its members. The organization includes such distinguished names as actors Warren Mitchell and Paul Eddington. Launched in September 1984, it quickly had an impact. Philip Morris, anticipating trouble, backed out of sponsoring *Raffles*, a play at the Watford Palace Theatre. Imperial Tobacco paradoxically warned that it would pull out of arts sponsorship if the campaign took off – exactly what the actors wanted! The organization received important backing when Sir Roy Shaw, secretary-general of the Arts Council from 1975 to 1983, joined. Tobacco companies spend an estimated £1.25 million on arts sponsorship each year.

Since December 1985 there has been a renewed assault in Parliament on smoking, designed to coincide with the negotiations for new agreements with the tobacco industry on advertising and sports sponsorship. Two new bills were introduced by Labour back-benchers Laurie Pavitt and Roger Sims. Neither had the remotest chance of reaching the statute book but both were good propaganda: Laurie Pavitt's bill would ban tobacco advertising, while Roger Sims's would phase out sports sponsorship by the tobacco industry. Another MP introduced a Private Members' bill to ban the sale of tobacco or any tobacco product to anyone under sixteen – a bill aimed at the sale of Skoal Bandits to youngsters. Nearly 100 MPs signed a Commons motion calling on the government to impose effective restrictions on its sale and promotion.

One argument the tobacco companies fall back on time and time again is that 'there is no evidence that sponsoring events leads to an increase in people smoking or to young people taking up smoking'. One might echo the words of many advertising executives, who see this claim as nonsense. The evidence that has been gathered shows that cigarette companies that sponsor events do make an impact on the minds of young people, which can only encourage them to smoke. Confidential figures inside the industry apparently have led to the conclusion that advertising, and that would include sponsorship, does have a 'highly significant influence on primary demand'.

A survey by the Addiction Research Unit at London's Institute of Psychiatry questioned 880 children soon after a snooker championship sponsored by Benson and Hedges had received twenty-eight hours of television coverage. It found that 70 per cent of the child smokers said they preferred Benson and Hedges. Another survey in early 1965 carried out at a girls comprehensive school in an inner-city area in the south of England showed that 91 per cent of the pupils who smoked had a preference for one particular type of cigarette; 80 per cent of these preferred Benson and Hedges. Benson and Hedges had been one of two companies which had recently sponsored snooker tournaments on television. The seduction of children by the tobacco companies should be of paramount concern to all those interested in the future.

11 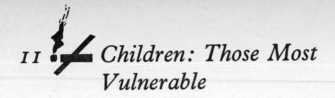 Children: Those Most Vulnerable

The influence of advertising and sponsorship on children is particularly important. It is often said that it is really youngsters that tobacco companies are after, because once hooked they will probably be smokers for life.

One in three people who become regular smokers started before they were nine. Even children who smoke one cigarette a week regularly are placing themselves in a vulnerable position so far as becoming a regular smoker later is concerned. Most children who regularly smoke one cigarette a week ultimately become habitual smokers, and the earlier an adult started smoking as a child the more likely he is to die as a result of the habit.[24]

There have been many surveys to try to find out why children take up smoking. The fact that children see advertisements for cigarettes does not help, nor does the fact that they can often buy cigarettes at tobacconists, even though it is illegal for a tobacconist to sell them to children. However, peer-group pressure is probably one of the strongest motivating forces. Children do not understand the strongly addictive nature of smoking. The Royal College of Physicians report on smoking in 1971 attempted to analyse the sort of boys who take up smoking. It identified them as tending to be less successful at work and games. They felt smoking gave them an aura of toughness and precocity.

In Britain in 1982 children aged eleven to sixteen spent £60 million on smoking. By 1984 the figure had reached £90 million. In 1982 a survey of 15,000 children in Tyne and Wear showed that a quarter of sixteen-year-olds were smoking regularly and among nineteen-year-olds 28 per cent were regular smokers.[25] Many of them had fixed views about what they saw as the benefits of smoking. Nearly a quarter of those interviewed thought that smoking helped to keep down their weight and 40 per cent thought it calmed their nerves. It is astonishing how young some children start their smoking habit. Surveys have shown that about 5 to 6 per cent of eleven- and twelve-year-old boys smoke more than forty cigarettes a week. Even more astonishingly, a quarter of ten- to twelve-year-olds said they had their first cigarette with their parents or were given it by their parents. The popularity of low-tar cigarettes could paradoxically be a bad thing, because they make the initial physical effects of smoking less unpleasant for children and therefore might make it easier for children to take up the habit regularly.

In 1981 a survey in Ireland found that there was a high level of smoking among school children. Smoking among girls in particular had increased over the previous decade from 18 per cent to 26 per cent. In this survey more than half the children said they would like to stop, not for health reasons but because they were worried about the cost of smoking and its effect on sporting performance.[26]

A survey by the Office of Population Censuses and Surveys in 1982 showed that about one in five children smoked, and nearly one in ten were regular smokers.[27] The regular smokers smoked on average about fifty cigarettes a week. Many smokers deluded themselves into believing they were not hooked. Only 65 per cent of them said they expected to be regular smokers when they left school. A similar survey two years later showed the situation had not improved. This survey made the point that child smokers seem to have a powerful emotional bond with the cigarette habit, forged under the special conditions of adolescence.

The figures from various surveys show a steady pattern. The ease with which children get hold of cigarettes is clearly demonstrated by surveys in various parts of England and Wales. In one survey, of fifty shops investigated forty-three sold cigarettes to children who were obviously younger than sixteen.[28] Some shopkeepers warned children that they were breaking the law in buying cigarettes and that they 'had better look out for policemen' on leaving the shop. But few tobacconists are caught and prosecuted. Between 1972 and 1977 prosecutions for breaches of this law averaged only twenty a year. A survey in 1983 by an Exeter GP of thirty-seven local shops found that twenty-eight of them sold cigarettes to children. The sales people said they did not understand the law. Another survey in Bristol showed that only nine out of 100 shops refused to sell cigarettes to children.

In June 1984 the junior health minister, John Patten, met retail organizations to tell them of his plans to issue guidelines to shopkeepers to prevent widespread abuse of the law which forbids them to sell cigarettes to children under sixteen. It is said that 88 per cent of children who smoke buy their cigarettes in shops.

There is strong support among the public for raising the age at which cigarettes can be bought from sixteen to eighteen. This was one of the conclusions in a survey conducted by the Office of Population Censuses and Surveys, which found that 65 per cent of a group of 4,000 people – both smokers and non-smokers – agreed that the legal age should be raised to eighteen.

So poorly is the law understood that in 1985 one local authority in Devon even found itself breaking the law indirectly by providing cigarettes to some of the children under sixteen in its care. The local authority used to stop the cost of the cigarettes the children smoked out of their £2 a week pocket money. It was thought this would help them understand that smoking was an expensive habit and encourage them to give up. Asked why smoking was allowed in children's homes at all, a council spokesman said that if they banned smoking it would just lead to children stealing cigarettes and smoking in secret.

Tobacconists do not always sell cigarettes to children due to ignorance of the law. Like the tobacco companies, they have a vested interest in selling to children. In January 1985 the tobacconists' trade paper reported that retailers were angry about an anti-smoking film made for children. It quoted Mr Harry Tipple of the Retail Confectioners and Tobacconists Association as saying that retailers were not against giving information to children in principle, 'but anything that restricts freedom of choice is bad ... I shall want to know the contents in more detail but I don't like it already because I believe they should ask the parents' permission.'

In the past few years there have been some valiant official attempts to persuade children not to smoke. A health education programme involving the children's hero Superman was designed for seven- to eleven-year-olds and ran from 1980 to 1983. The hero battled with a degenerate 'pusher' of cigarettes called Nick O'Teen. This programme included a scheme where children could write requesting packs of material including signed certificates testifying to their personal commitment against smoking. As a result of the 1981 media campaign 600,000 wrote to the Health Education Council. In the 1970s the Health Education Council and the Schools Council developed national curriculum projects – six were published between 1977 and 1983. It is thought that up to a million children each year have been influenced by the project designed for five- to thirteen-year-olds.

There is some firm evidence that these sorts of projects do work. A study which followed 6,000 children during their school career found that more boys and girls smoked if they had attended a school with no anti-smoking health education. One school in Manchester even set up a 'stop smoking' clinic for children at school. The clinic met once a week during the lunch hour and was meant to give children help in stopping smoking in a group situation.

However, there is still a distinct impression that the government is being half-hearted about the effort it devotes to educating children not to smoke. Experts cite one recent action by the education secretary, Sir Keith Joseph: in November 1983 he appointed a representative from the tobacco industry to serve on a committee which was designed to advise the government on what is taught in schools. The twenty-three members of the Curriculum Development Committee included the personnel manager of the tobacco manufacturer John Player!

Although it is true to say that the British government's commitment against smoking has been half-hearted, it has provided limited funds for anti-smoking organizations from time to time. As recently as December 1985 it provided £1 million for a test advertising campaign in certain areas to discourage teenagers from smoking and pledged that if it were judged a success, it would spend a further £5 million to bring the anti-smoking message into every household in the country. This was prompted partly by figures showing a rise in the number of youngsters smoking. A survey by the Office of Population Censuses and Surveys published in December 1985 showed that in certain groups smoking was up. The figures were based on 9,000 pupils at 300 schools, and showed that 45 per cent of girls aged sixteen smoke. It showed that although boys experiment with smoking at an earlier age than girls, girls catch up and possibly overtake boys in their fourth secondary-school year.

There are those who claim that the way the tobacco companies try to influence young people to smoke is immoral. The same is true of the way the industry exploits the Third World.

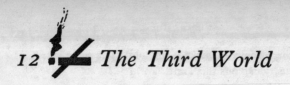

While it seems that in some developed countries the warnings are at last hitting home and that the incidence of smoking is declining, it is a different story in the Third World. The result is that world-wide the total sales of cigarettes have been increasing. World production of cigarettes increased from an annual average of 3,349 billion between 1968 and 1972 to 4,126 billion in 1977, much of the increase being in the Third World. In the last twenty years, tobacco production by Third World countries has dramatically increased. In the 1960s, Third World countries contributed about 17 per cent of the world's production of tobacco. By 1976 their contribution had reached 40 per cent. Of the top ten producers, five are in the Third World: China, India, Brazil, South Korea and Indonesia. While the output of cigarettes from 1968 to 1976 increased in Britain by an average of 1.7 per cent and by 3.3 per cent in America, in Indonesia it increased by over 12 per cent, in Nigeria by 10 per cent and in Kenya by 8 per cent.

Between 1965 and 1975 the world consumption of cigarettes rose by about 3 to 4 per cent a year. Although it has slowed down since then in the developed world, in the developing world it has continued to rise by 5 per cent a year. In the last few years growth has been rather less steep, partly because of the world-wide recession, retail price increases and the intensification of anti-smoking campaigns. Adverse weather conditions have also affected the growing of tobacco in certain countries.

While governments in the developed world have started to come to grips with smoking, albeit in a rather desultory fashion, in the majority of developing countries the tobacco companies are still exploiting ignorance, poverty and gullibility among the population to promote smoking and swell their profits. The companies recognize that there is still a big potential for growth in the developing world. It is estimated that each Third World smoker consumes an average of only 300 cigarettes a year compared with the average Western smoker's 2,500. The World Health Organization suggests that these figures show there is still time for action to prevent the smoking holocaust which has affected the West. However, the smoking-linked diseases are already increasing remorselessly in the developing world. At one of the largest cancer hospitals in São Paulo, for example, over the past forty years lung-cancer deaths have nearly trebled among men aged forty to forty-nine; they have increased nearly seven times in men aged between fifty and fifty-nine, and nearly nine times in men aged between sixty and sixty-nine. Lung cancer is the third most common cancer among men in Brazil and is rapidly approaching the number one position. In India, lung-cancer deaths in smokers are well over eight times those in non-smokers. World-wide it is estimated that a million people a year are now developing cigarette-linked tumours.

The World Health Organization has launched a campaign to convince governments that cancer is a growing problem in developing countries. Lung-cancer mortality is growing as a result of what the WHO calls 'the energetic expansion of sales of high-nicotine cigarettes in developing countries'. An article in the *Lancet* in January 1984 suggested that in previous centuries the arrival of cholera and the plague from the Orient brought fear and trembling to the citizens of this country. But now it is the developing countries that should stand in fear of the plague of the cigarette, which tobacco companies based in Britain are exporting to the Third World. The article criticized Britain for doing practically nothing to help the Third World tackle its smoking problem. Indeed, between 1974 and 1979 Britain actually gave £3.5 million to four Commonwealth countries for the *development* of their tobacco industries. Norway and Sweden, in contrast, give substantial sums to the International Union against Cancer and the World Health Organization for anti-smoking programmes. The article concluded,

These companies are causing a new form of Third World slavery, which is yearly killing tens of thousands who die unaware of the risks they have been taking. Wilberforce succeeded after forty years. We shall have to take stronger action if, with regard to smoking, we are to emulate his achievement.

The World Health Organization has warned of the way the cigarette companies react whenever they feel themselves threatened in a particular country. They immediately start long-drawn-out nego-tiations with the health authorities with a view to creating confusion and buying time to prevent effective action to control smoking.

Statistics are being poured out almost daily about the impact of smoking throughout the world. Just a few will suffice to demonstrate how much it is a global problem.[29] In Pakistan 120,000 acres of land are given over to growing tobacco. Cigarette consumption is increasing at 8 per cent a year. Lung cancer in Pakistan is now the most common form of cancer among men. In Sri Lanka cigarette consumption has been increasing by nearly 8 per cent a year. In Thailand 20 per cent of the population over ten are smokers. Twenty per cent of individual income is spent on smoking. In Katmandu, 78 per cent of men smoke and 80 per cent of men in urban Senegal. In Lagos 72 per cent of medical students smoke, and 39 per cent of doctors in Bangladesh. In the last eleven years the incidence of lung cancer among the Bantu in the Natal in South Africa has increased sixfold.

Growth rates in cigarette markets in developed and developing countries 1975–84 (percentages)

Country	1975–80	1980–84
Developed		
Austria	+1.8	0.0
Germany	+0.5	−1.5
USA	+0.5	−0.5
UK	−1.8	−3.4
Developing		
Brazil	+4.1	−2.1
Malaysia	+4.7	+4.8
India	+5.6	+3.6
Pakistan	+6.1	+1.9

Source: Tobacco Advisory Council (unpublished figures)

In many of these developing countries tobacco is not just smoked in cigarettes. Other ways of absorbing the nicotine have evolved, many of them carrying their own particular dangers. In Pakistan tobacco is smoked through the hookah, and chewed as *pan*, which contains tobacco and betel nut; it is used also as a plug in the mouth (*niswar*) or smoked in the form of *bidi*. In India some people smoke *chuttas*, or coarse cheroots, with the lighted end inside their mouths. A ten-year study of over 10,000 people living in the Srikakulam district of India showed that more women chew tobacco than men and they have a higher death-rate than those who did not use tobacco.

One of the worrying aspects of Third World smoking is that the cigarettes marketed in these countries tend to have a much higher tar content than cigarettes sold in the West. In Pakistan, for example, two of the most popular brands, Capstan and Morven, each have a yield of 29 mg tar per cigarette. Tar concentrations for a range of popular cigarettes sold in the United Kingdom and in Australia in 1981 never exceeded 19 mg tar per cigarette. By contrast, the same cigarettes sold in Singapore give tar yields of 19 to 33 mg per cigarette. Even the brands with the lowest available tar yield would barely be described as 'middle tar' in the UK, although tobacco companies do claim that some reductions in tar and nicotine yields in developing countries are being made.

Apart from the type of cigarettes sold, the way they are promoted is far more aggressive than is allowed in the West, and compared with what the West is used to many of the advertisements in the developing world seem positively immoral. The 1983 Royal College of Physicians report, *Health or Smoking*, drew attention to the advertising policies of the tobacco companies.

In countries where health education and the awareness of the dangers of smoking are virtually non-existent, where adult literacy is low, where there is much less consumer advertising than in the West and where the desire to copy Western habits is all too apparent, even a relatively small expenditure on advertising can be effective, not least in simply promoting the idea and desirability of smoking.

Even the names which have been used for cigarette brands in the last few years show the blatant disregard the companies have for the facts about smoking. One leading brand of cigarette in Africa was called 'Life'. In Egypt, Taiwan, Bangladesh and Uganda names have been chosen for cigarettes which imply exactly the opposite of what cigarettes really stand for – names like 'Cleopatra', 'Nefertiti', 'Long Life', 'New Paradise', 'Champion' and 'Sportsman'.

In Argentina cigarette advertising takes up 20 per cent of all television advertising time. The advertisements portray young men surrounded by admiring girls and are obviously aimed at the younger generation. The Argentinian health ministry admits that 'while such advertising is supposed to be for brand support, it is in fact intended to attract the young generation'.

Indeed, the claim by tobacco manufacturers that advertising is not intended to encourage people to smoke but just to switch brands is easily invalidated by the fact that in Kenya British American Tobacco had a monopoly on cigarettes until the late 1970s, yet it was the country's fourth largest commercial advertiser. The market there is growing by 8 per cent a year. Kenya is a good illustration of how ruthless and aggressive cigarette advertising can be. The mobile cinema is used extensively, and advertisements emphasize the supposed link between cigarettes and success. The advertisement for Sportsman cigarettes depicts an individual in four 'successful' situations: choosing the best vegetables at the market, the best suit at the tailors, the winning horse at the races and buying Sportsman cigarettes. This form of advertising is, of course, no longer permitted in the West. There are no health warnings on cigarette packets and people have no information about the dangers of smoking. In 1974 and 1978 the World Health Organization recommended, among other things, government control of marketing. It has not happened in Kenya.

Tobacco is, of course, a major crop in many developing countries and many hundreds of thousands of people depend on it for their livelihood. Governments depend on the sale of cigarettes for revenue and it provides valuable foreign exchange. In Zimbabwe, for example, tobacco is the nation's largest employer. It helps support 17,000 tobacco farmers. In Malawi 100,000 families rely on cash income from tobacco. In Tanzania tobacco provides income for about 370,000 people – some 2 per cent of the population. In the south of Brazil there are 115,000 tobacco farmers and a further 650,000 people directly dependent on tobacco. The tobacco crop yields far higher returns than any of the major food crops.

World export of tobacco in 1979–81 averaged $4,000 million, of which nearly half accrued to developing countries. In some ways the tobacco giants have many of the developing countries in their grip. It is the companies who set up the tobacco farmer in business, helping him to buy his equipment and a curing barn. They provide free tobacco seed and provide fertilizer and insecticide at cost price. In his book *The Smoke Ring* Peter Taylor makes it clear that even if a country wanted to wean its people off growing tobacco they could not afford to do so. To match the companies' loans and to subsidize the price, the price the farmer would be paid for his food crop would cost too much – the countries do not have the resources of the big tobacco giants.

Yet while the tobacco companies reap huge profits from tobacco, many of the people in the Third World countries are starving. A letter in the *Guardian* asked recently what proportion of the profits from the sale of these cigarettes was returned to these countries by the companies as a contribution to famine relief?

One of the most serious aspects of the development of tobacco growing in Third World countries is the effect it has on forests. Growers need wood to cure, or dry, the tobacco leaves after harvesting. It is estimated that one in eight of all trees felled throughout the world is used for flue-curing tobacco. The tobacco leaf is cured by exposing it to a constant temperature of 160°F for a week. It has been estimated that 150 large trees are needed to cure just one acre of tobacco. In Brazil, for example, the 100,000 tobacco farmers of Rio Grande do Sul are thought to need the wood of six million trees.

While huge areas of forest have been stripped to provide wood for curing, some 80 per cent of the energy is wasted. The tobacco companies try to encourage replacement tree planting, but as their profits from the sale of tobacco increase, farmers are able to buy increasingly expensive fuel from outside the area, so there is little incentive for them to plant trees. In Kenya the annual tobacco production requires the felling of some 5,000 to 8,000 hectares of forest each year. At present rates of felling there may be no trees left in Kenya by the year 2000. The slopes on the sides of the Kunati valley near Mount Kenya are now completely bare. Farmers have tried to grow maize on the hillsides but heavy rains wash away the soil, plants and all. The topsoil has been eroded in some places, and rocks and boulders are already being washed down towards the fertile fields below. Although British American Tobacco provides eucalyptus seedlings, deforestation happens much faster than the new trees can grow in the bare hillside soil. All this is a relatively new phenomenon. There was little tobacco-leaf production in Kenya before 1973. In

Tanzania it is estimated that in the last twenty years 120,000 tons of flue-cured tobacco have been produced, which has decimated 240,000 hectares of forest.

The tobacco industry is concerned about the way its critics are concentrating their attention on the industry's activities in the Third World. The stand they have adopted can be judged by a memorandum produced for the international tobacco industry after the fourth World Conference on Smoking and Health in 1979, which included the following statement:

We must try to stop the development towards a Third World commitment against tobacco. We must try to get all, or at least a substantial part of, Third World countries committed to our cause. We must try to influence official FAO and UNCTAD policy to take a pro-tobacco stand. We must try to mitigate the impact of the World Health Organization, by pushing them into a more objective and neutral position.

The Royal College of Physicians report commented:

There can be no doubt that smoking in developing countries is an adversarial problem, and that only the most determined action by those concerned to promote health will succeed in curbing the activities of the international tobacco industry ... The international tobacco industry can be expected to oppose and hinder efforts to reduce smoking. In doing so it will be directly responsible for fostering the deaths of thousands in the twentieth century's most avoidable epidemic.

The first Third World country where cigarette smoking was declared to be the leading avoidable cause of death by the World Health Organization was Brazil. In 1979 ischaemic heart disease in Brazil caused 90,000 deaths – much of which can be attributed to smoking. Up to 20,000 cancer deaths a year are due to smoking. The incidence of low-birth-weight babies is doubled in women who smoke. Brazil has a high rate of infant mortality – seventy-two deaths per 1,000 live births – and low birth-weight is a major factor. These figures mean that in 1984 smoking may have killed some 40,000 adults and 40,000 babies. Yet despite this appalling cost, smoking in Brazil is on the increase and the government derives just over 11 per cent of its tax revenue from cigarettes. Cigarettes are promoted on Brazilian television with blatant disregard for the dangers they pose. Every effort is made to make smoking seem attractive to young people. Advertisements for

Hollywood cigarettes, for example, have included shots of attractive young people riding in dune buggies over the sand, driving fast, expensive cars and so on. The cigarettes are given away at sponsored events by beautiful girls in miniskirts. Yet the chairman and managing director of the company which dominates the Brazilian market was quoted as saying that, so far as promotion is concerned, the managers in developing countries 'are aware that local practice should not be incompatible with promotional standards in the industrialized nations'.

Not all Third World countries have had the wool pulled over their eyes by the tobacco companies and some are fighting back. In January 1983 the Sudanese government brought in a law which banned all cigarette advertising and required health warnings to be printed on packets. It also passed an act forbidding smoking in public places and on public transport. Following the ban on advertising the tobacco companies asked for a six-month postponement while they made preparations. Once the ban was in force Philip Morris simply removed the cigarette packets from their Marlboro advertisements and substituted cigarette lighters!

In Malaysia the death toll from smoking continues to rise. There the best-selling cigarette is Benson and Hedges. In 1983 the brand contained 31 mg tar per cigarette, compared with only 17 mg in the equivalent cigarette in Britain. The Malaysian Tobacco Corporation, a subsidiary of British American Tobacco, which makes Benson and Hedges, says it will reduce tar and nicotine in cigarettes made locally 'if and when there is a shift in preference toward lower tar and nicotine cigarettes'. Here too the government has acted. In 1982 it banned cigarette advertising on radio and television, prohibited smoking in all government offices and encouraged state governments to forbid bill-board advertising. Its efforts paid off. Two years later in 1984 the Malaysian Medical Association reported that for the first time there had been a decline in the Malaysian cigarette market. Profits for the two biggest tobacco companies had fallen by 10 per cent in one case and 20 per cent in the other.

In Mexico a new general-health law will, it is hoped, cut cigarette consumption by 15 per cent within one year. The legislation covers such things as the sale of cigarettes to minors and health warnings on cigarette packets.

The country where smoking is more prevalent than anywhere else is China. There 700 billion cigarettes are sold every year – 100 billion more than in the United States. China has 200 million smokers, but the government is stepping up its efforts to persuade people not to smoke. The Central Patriotic Health Campaign and the Ministry of Public Health issued a circular calling for smoking to be banned or restricted in public places, and asking all cigarette factories to label their products with a health hazard warning. However, they have a big fight ahead. At least one Chinese factory has a label touting its brands as 'healthy cigarettes'.

In the last two years the world market has not been strong, partly due to the anti-smoking pressure groups and also because of deteriorating real incomes. An international commodity report published in October 1985 pointed out that because of the sluggish market, prices will not rise dramatically in the next year or so. Indeed there will be increased competition among the tobacco manufacturers for their market share. Turkey abolished its export tax on tobacco leaf in 1983, and similarly the United States, in an attempt to improve competitiveness on international markets, substantially modified its tobacco production and price-support policies in 1983. It warned that other countries were likely to embark on or strengthen similar measures in order to improve their market position.

Despite the apparently relentless progress of the tobacco industry in influencing the Third World, a new force is now coming to the fore in the West, which could dramatically change the climate of opinion surrounding smoking and represent the biggest challenge yet to the tobacco giants: the voice of the non-smoker.

13 The Power of the Non-Smoker

The knowledge that smoking can damage your health has been recognized now for over thirty years, and millions of people have given up smoking because of it. Governments have formulated policies, without much conviction it must be said, in an effort to stem the death toll without affecting too markedly the revenue they derive from cigarettes. And while the situation is improving in certain advanced countries, in the Third World it is getting worse because of what can only be described as ruthless exploitation of people's ignorance and weaknesses by the international tobacco companies.

However, a new force is slowly coming to the fore, which has already had a marked affect on the public acceptability of smoking and which could in the long run do more to turn people against tobacco than anything else that has been tried. For the first time the voice of the *non*-smoker is being heard, protesting not just that smoking is unpleasant or even that it infringes a person's right to breathe fresh air – both of which are perfectly valid objections – but also that having to breathe other people's smoke is now accepted as a health hazard. The non-smokers' right to health is being infringed and that is already bringing about a revolution in public attitudes towards whether smoking is acceptable behaviour or not. There is growing evidence that it is not. Non-smokers forced to breathe other people's smoke are at risk, and their attitude is increasingly likely to drive smoking behind closed doors so that it becomes, in the famous words of one of Britain's most notable chief medical officers, Sir George Godber, something which is only acceptable when it is done by consenting adults in private. The 1977 Royal College of Physicians report *Smoking or Health* urged a change in public attitudes so that smoking would become unusual in public places and special provision would have to be made for those who wish to smoke.

It is now recognized that non-smokers who breathe other people's smoke can have a respiratory disease aggravated, children can be harmed, and there is even evidence that passive, or forced, smoking, as it is called, can lead to life-threatening disorders like lung cancer. As early as 1970 ten bills were introduced in America at local level to restrict smoking in public places. By 1980 there were nearly 200. By 1980, forty-six states had some form of state or local laws banning or restricting smoking.

The industry recognizes the issue of passive smoking as of fundamental importance. In 1978 a survey warned the industry that not only did nine out of ten Americans believe smoking was hazardous to health, but most thought that passive smoking was a health hazard too. In addition, most of those questioned wanted separate smoking areas in public places and what is more, most said they would give their political support to a candidate who favoured a ban on smoking in public places.

A burning cigarette produces two kinds of smoke: that which is drawn through the cigarette into the smoker's lungs and then exhaled is called mainstream smoke; the smoke which billows into the room directly from the burning tip is called sidestream smoke. Because it has not passed through the cigarette, sidestream smoke is unfiltered and contains a greater concentration of unpleasant chemicals. There is, for example, 2.7 times as much nicotine in this unfiltered smoke, 2.5 times as much carbon monoxide, 73 times as much ammonia and 3.4 times as much of the carcinogen benzo-a-pyrene. By the time this smoke is breathed in by the passive smoker it has been diluted by the air in the room but it is still a health hazard.

In 1982 the average cigarette in the UK yielded 16 to 17 mg of carbon monoxide in mainstream smoke and about 40 mg in the sidestream. Measurements of various kinds of air show that smoke-free air contains about 2 ppm (parts per million) of carbon monoxide. At parties the carbon-monoxide concentration can go up to 7 to 9 ppm. In a conference room where delegates smoke the air can contain up to 33 ppm of carbon monoxide and smoking in a car can give as much as 112 ppm. In a room where there is good ventilation there are usually 3 ppm carbon monoxide when smokers are not present and 10 ppm when they are. With 10 ppm carbon monoxide in a room the amount of carboxyhaemoglobin in the blood of non-smokers might rise to 2 per cent. After exposure to 38 ppm carbon monoxide for over an hour the increase of carboxyhaemoglobin is about equal to that produced by smoking one cigarette.

Passive smoking can irritate the eyes – an effect due to the acrolein in the smoke – and it can also result in irritation of the throat, a cough and can cause headache. The problem can be particularly acute at work where non-smokers have no option but to stay in a smoky environment. Surveys have shown that non-smokers are inconvenienced by tobacco smokers at work. While better ventilation can help, modern recirculating systems do not filter out carbon monoxide. People exposed to increased levels of carbon monoxide clearly cannot work as well as those breathing ordinary air. Tests have shown that exercise is performed less efficiently, the time taken to reach exhaustion is less, there is a greater increase in heart rate and the effect of this is particularly noticeable in older people. Volunteers exercising in a smoky atmosphere showed a small decrease in lung function.

There is evidence that people who breathe other people's smoke regularly are also at increased risk of developing lung cancer. When doctors compared the lung cancer rates of non-smokers married to smokers and non-smokers, they found that those married to smokers and therefore exposed frequently to smoky atmospheres showed an increased tendency to develop lung cancer. It has also been shown statistically that the amount of nicotine and tar inhaled by passive smoking could theoretically increase lung cancer in non-smokers by about 10 to 20 per cent.

To put the risk of passive smoking into proportion, it is possible to compare it with other hazards which apparently cause concern. It has been estimated that the risk of getting lung cancer from passive smoking is fifty times greater than the risk of working in an office building where there is asbestos in the structure, yet as Sir Richard Doll has pointed out, companies have spent millions over the past few years removing asbestos from workplaces, even though that process itself, unless precautions are very strictly observed, can create a problem. Looked at from another point of view, the risk of getting cancer from passive smoking is over 100 times greater than the risk to the general population from all cancers which might be caused by the operation of the nuclear industry, over which a great deal of fuss has been made by the anti-nuclear lobby. The lobby argues that nuclear hazards should not be compared with smoking because people can choose for themselves whether they smoke or not, whereas people have no choice over the development of the nuclear industry. The fact is that people have little choice over passive smoking – a strong argument for further restrictions on smoking in public places.

Let us take a closer look at some of the studies which have revealed the risk of passive smoking. A study in Japan quoted in the 1983 Royal College of Physicians report compared the risk of lung cancer run by non-smoking wives whose husbands smoked twenty cigarettes a day or more with the risk run by those wives whose husbands did not smoke. The wives of the smokers were more than twice as likely to develop lung cancer. For the wives whose husbands smoked fewer than twenty a day the risk went down to 1.6 times. Other studies have confirmed this. As the RCP report put it, 'Overall ... results are consistent with a 50 per cent increase in lung cancer in the non-smoking wives of husbands who smoke.'

A Japanese professor writing to the *Lancet* in 1984 revealed that apart from having an increased risk of lung cancer, wives of men who smoked were also at increased risk of cancer of the paranasal sinuses. An American research report from the National Institute of Environmental Health Sciences has shown that the risk of developing leukaemia rises nearly seven times among those people who have lived with three or more people who smoked. The risk of breast cancer rises 3.3 times and the risk of cervical cancer rises 3.4 times.

A study from the US Environmental Protection Agency estimates that from 500 to 5,000 lung-cancer deaths in America among non-smokers are due to passive smoking, and says that tobacco smoke is the country's most dangerous carcinogen. (The second most dangerous common airborne carcinogen is coke oven gas, which is implicated in up to 160 lung-cancer deaths a year.)

Passive smokers also have raised nicotine levels. About half the non-smokers in cities have raised nicotine levels in their blood, and most have nicotine in their urine. A study by Dr Michael Russell of the Addiction Research Unit at the Institute of Psychiatry in London says that urban non-smokers and children whose parents smoked had measurable levels of nicotine in their bodies, which averaged about 0.5 per cent of the levels found in smokers. 'If the risks of diseases caused by smoking are related to dose in a linear fashion, as they appear to be, the intake from passive smoking could be causing about 1,000 smoke-related deaths a year among non-smokers in Britain.'

In some countries the courts are now beginning to accept that passive smoking is a health hazard. In Sweden a few years ago a 55-year-old woman who died of lung cancer had her illness classified as an industrial injury because her colleagues at work smoked. She had worked for twenty years in a drawing office with six heavy smokers. The ventilation had been bad and opening windows was not allowed. The Health Insurance Court of southern Sweden heard evidence from a medical expert arguing that the lung cancer may have been caused by passive smoking and three of the four other expert witnesses agreed.

Perhaps concern should be greatest for the plight of children exposed to passive smoking in the home, because it is clear from research that even from a young age, children's health can be adversely affected if they are constantly exposed to their parents' smoking habits. One survey of children exposed to a smoky atmosphere found that during a period of five years the lung function of non-smoking children with mothers who smoked developed at only 93 per cent of the rate at which that of non-smoking children with non-smoking mothers developed.[30] The scientists who conducted this survey suggest that the loss in lung capacity might mean that the children could develop obstructive-airways disease in later life.

Another study showed that children who were exposed to smoke at home tended to have an increased incidence of middle-ear infections.[31] If they were exposed to smoke from two or more smokers their risk of ear infections rose threefold. Infections like this are important because they can cause hearing loss and associated language and learning difficulties.

Children exposed to a smoky atmosphere have more respiratory symptoms and are more prone to respiratory infections than children of non-smokers. This is especially noticeable in the first year of life, when pneumonia and bronchitis are more than twice as common in infants whose parents smoke than in those of non-smoking parents. Maternal smoking habits are more important than paternal and the effect diminishes with age, showing the importance of close physical contact.

Children who suffer from these infections show clear evidence of impaired lung function at five years of age, and children of smoking parents are on average up to 1 cm shorter than other children at primary school. According to research quoted in the 1983 Royal College of Physicians report, by the age of eleven children whose parents smoke may be as much as six months behind their contemporaries whose parents do not smoke in such subjects as reading comprehension and mathematics.

One large study of older children in the north of England found that they tended to report more coughs if their parents smoked compared with children whose parents did not smoke. Of those boys under eleven with parents who did not smoke 35 per cent said they had 'a lot of coughs'. For those boys with one parent who smoked the figure increased to 42 per cent, and 48 per cent of boys with both parents who smoked complained of having a lot of coughs. It was a similar story with girls.

Tests on babies exposed to smoke in the home show alarming results. Their urine and saliva can contain levels of nicotine and the nicotine metabolite, cotinine, which are within the range found in light smokers. It is not only the air babies breathe which gives them a dose of nicotine. Breast-feeding mothers who smoke also pass over nicotine in their milk.

By measuring the amount of cotinine in the saliva of children it is possible to express their exposure to tobacco smoke in terms of the number of cigarettes they would have to smoke to reach those levels. Hence in a family where the father smokes it is as if the child himself smoked thirty cigarettes a year. If the mother smokes, it is equivalent to the child having fifty cigarettes a year (or one a week), and if both parents smoke, the equivalent smoking rate for the child would be eighty a year. Experts from the Institute of Psychiatry Addiction Research Unit suggest that 'this unsolicited burden may be prolonged throughout childhood and poses a definite risk to health'.

In the last few years there have been moves to limit smoking in public places, not only because it is a health hazard but also because of the nuisance of other people's smoke. Smoking has been curtailed in public transport and there have also been pressures on employers to do something about limiting areas where people can smoke at work. Once again it is the man in the street who has led the way, with the government apparently being pulled reluctantly along behind. In

November 1967 the minister of health was asked in Parliament about restrictions on smoking in public places. He said then, 'There is some reluctance to impose further restrictions on smoking which may prove unpopular with the public.' Yet the *Social Survey* even then found that only a minority – some 40 per cent – of the public opposed a ban on smoking in buses and only one in five objected to an increase in non-smoking compartments in trains. Later surveys showed that the public as a whole is sympathetic to increasing non-smoking facilities. A survey in 1976 showed that nearly three-quarters of those questioned favoured restrictions on smoking in cinemas, aeroplanes, buses, hospitals and restaurants. In the same year the Institute of Professional Civil Servants passed a resolution asserting the rights of their members to have non-smoking office accommodation. A survey in 1983 conducted by the Office of Population Censuses and Surveys covering 3,764 smokers and non-smokers found that there was very strong support for the right of non-smokers to enjoy smoke-free air at work, although much less support for a total ban on smoking in the workplace. There was again wide support for a ban on smoking in many, though not all, public places. The survey showed that among non-smokers, nearly a third said they were frequently bothered by smoke and a further 42 per cent said they were occasionally bothered by it. Yet despite this, less than a quarter protested about it. A fifth of non-smokers said they avoided places where they knew there would be smoke. Authorities are not altogether immune to the complaints of those who hate other people's smoke – in 1983 a woman was excused jury service at the Old Bailey because she was unwilling to endure other jurors smoking in the jury room.

However, if the government in Britain is largely indifferent to the pleas of non-smokers who want to breathe fresh air, in America it is a different story. Since the early 1970s, various anti-smoking groups have tried to ban smoking in public places. A mechanism exists there by which people can enact legislation themselves in a referendum at certain times if sufficient numbers vote in favour of particular propositions. Several attempts have been made in various states to try to ban smoking in public places this way. Each time such a proposition threatened, the tobacco industry spent huge sums of money trying to persuade people not to support it, claiming that their basic freedoms were at stake. The industry usually won, until a proposition was mooted in San Francisco in 1983, which required all employers to adopt a written policy to accommodate smokers and non-smokers in the workplace. The industry fought it on the grounds that it would breed conflict, drive people apart and set friend against friend, and also that once again it was an example of too much government. However, this time the industry lost, despite the money it spent on its campaign. In 1983 the mayor of San Francisco, Dianne Feinstein, signed into law a city ordnance regulating smoking in offices. It states that if smoking is permitted in an office, the employer must make accommodation for the preference of both non-smoking and smoking employees, but if the non-smokers are not happy with the arrangements, then smoking must be prohibited. It also called for every employer to produce their written smoking policy within three months.

The reaction from the Tobacco Institute of America was unsurprising: a spokesman said the ordnance was unnecessary, unenforceable and would lead to 'class discrimination, where anyone with a private office does not have to worry about the restriction but anyone who sits with others or where the public comes can have that privilege revoked'.[32] However, many companies did not wait to be dragooned into introducing consideration for the non-smokers in their offices. By 1983 one in three American companies had in-house rules protecting the rights of non-smoking employees. They had the right to insist on smoke-free places to work in.

Los Angeles soon joined San Francisco in approving local laws to control smoking at work. Employers in Los Angeles now have to provide separate areas for smokers and non-smokers at work. If no agreement can be reached on shared office space, non-smokers have to be given preference. Those employers who fail to protect non-smokers can receive a jail sentence of up to six months and a fine of up to $500.

Also in 1983 the US Department of Health Education and Welfare introduced regulations to protect its own non-smoking employees, which were later adopted by all government agencies. They make it clear that no worker should be required to work in an atmosphere containing tobacco smoke and this applies to conference rooms, classrooms and eating places. By 1983 some thirty states had passed legislation restricting smoking in public places. That year the Royal College of Physicians report pointed out the contrast between what had been done in America and the lack of firm action in Britain. It concluded, 'The non-smoking majority in the United Kingdom has every right to expect protection from the discomfort and danger of other people's cigarette smoke, as has already been largely achieved elsewhere.'

Other countries have also set an example. In Sweden in 1983 the Social and Welfare Board and the Board of Occupational Safety and Health were instructed by the government to draw up guidelines for limiting smoking in public places and work areas, and were given the equivalent of 85,000 American dollars to finance their work. In the Spanish parliament building smoking has been banned, not because of the danger to the lungs of those who sit in it, but in order to protect the frescos on the ceiling, which were found to be deteriorating as a result of exposure to tobacco fumes! In Moscow the Municipal Council has banned smoking in Red Square, the site of Lenin's tomb, and a similar ban has been introduced in Alexander Park, site of the tomb of the unknown soldier. The decision, it was said, was taken following requests from both Moscow citizens and visitors.

Britain lags a long way behind America in consideration for the rights of non-smokers. Of 100 companies surveyed by the Health Education Council and ASH in 1984, 45 per cent saw no advantage in having a smoking policy while 86 per cent saw disadvantages. Twenty-four per cent said it would infringe an individual's freedom of choice, and 16 per cent thought it would be harder to recruit staff with a smoking policy in force. None the less, facilities for non-smokers are improving all the time. There are now directories listing hotels, restaurants, guest houses and so on which make special provision for non-smokers, and many companies are beginning to recognize the rights of the non-smoker. In July 1985, to take just one example, the Cambridge University Press introduced a system whereby staff can smoke only in their own time and only in a small smoking room. They have to clock off to visit it and clock on again when they return. The ban on smoking was introduced with the backing of the staff.

The medical evidence is heavily in favour of the thesis that it is not only a nuisance but is potentially and actually harmful for non-smokers to have to breathe other people's smoke. In a country which prides itself on upholding the freedom of the individual it is about time the right of the individual *not* to have to breathe other people's smoke was as widely protected as the right of the individual to smoke if he wants to.

The freedom to do whatever one wants has never been absolute. Individual freedoms are already hedged around with qualifications often designed for the greater good of the community. People argued for a long time about an individual's right not to have to wear seat belts if he did not want to, but eventually seat-belt legislation was introduced and it has saved many lives. An individual may have a perfect right to place his life in danger by pursuing dangerous sports or hobbies, or not wearing a seat belt or smoking if he wishes. But does a married man with children or other dependants have a right to place his life in danger when his premature death would leave his wife and children bereft? Perhaps they too have a right to be protected from his foolishness.

One of the most iniquitous aspects of the smoking business is the way children and young people are being seduced into smoking by their constant exposure to advertisements for cigarettes. It is irresponsible of the tobacco industry to advertise cigarettes in such a way that children can be influenced, and of the government to allow it. For the last twenty years cigarette advertisements have been banned on television. There is no difference in principle between advertising on television and advertising anywhere else. If cigarette advertisements are unsuitable for television, they must also be unsuitable for magazines, newspapers and hoardings. On logical grounds then, there is a good case for the government to ban the advertising of cigarettes.

Even more pernicious than overt advertising is the way the cigarette companies have got around the ban on cigarette advertising on television by sponsorship – particularly of sports events which are shown on television. There is no justification for this. Most sponsored sports would not suffer if sponsorship by the tobacco industry were banned, because those events which have become popular on television like snooker and cricket would almost certainly survive thanks to other sponsors, should the tobacco industry be forced to withdraw. There is also something immoral about an industry which produces such a lethal product being allowed to associate it with a health-giving activity like sport.

The two priorities of the government, then, should be to ban the promotion of cigarettes by advertising and sponsorship. The evidence is that in those countries where this has happened sales have decreased, especially among the young, and it is the young who should represent the priority group. Once this has been achieved, it will rob the industry of the ability it exploits at the moment to invest cigarettes with an aura of respectability. The social climate will change so that smoking in public will become less acceptable. It would then be time for the government to further restrict smoking in public places. Already many public places have placed restrictions on smoking – theatres, some cinemas, some public transport and so on. The 'smoke-free zones' are expanding. Non-smokers are now in the majority. Indeed, over two thirds of the adult population are non-smokers. It is their wishes which should be respected. Smokers can always pursue their habit in the privacy of their own homes, assuming they can live with the fact that their smoke is probably having a deleterious effect on their own families. The government should also progressively increase the tax on cigarettes to deter smokers. As smoking declines, tobacco companies will be forced to diversify, as many are doing at the moment. As Third World countries see what is happening in the West they may be further encouraged to act against the tobacco companies before their own populations become as liable to decimation from smoking as those in the West.

Smoking is on the decline in the civilized world. If the pressure is maintained, the decline will be swift. In a hundred years' time people will hopefully look back at this century and regard the death and destruction we wrought on ourselves through smoking with the same horror we now experience when we look back to the era of the Black Death: a mixture of astonishment and pity for the plight of those who lived at that time.

Notes

1. Quoted in the *International Herald Tribune*, 24 and 25 November 1985.

2. *General Household Survey: Cigarette Smoking 1972–82*, OPCS Monitor, ref. GHS 83/3 (1983).

3. *General Household Survey: Cigarette Smoking 1972–84*, OPCS Monitor, ref. GHS 85/2 (1985).

4. *Tobacco Alert*, World Health Organization, ser. 1, vol. 2, no. 4 (December 1984).

5. A. C. McKennel and R. K. Thomas, *Adults' and Adolescents' Smoking Habits and Attitudes*, HMSO (1967).

6. C. McArthur et al., 'The Psychology of Smoking', *Journal of Abnormal and Social Psychology*, vol. 56, p. 267.

7. Quoted in a lecture by Sir Richard Doll, 'Medical Effects of Smoking – Problems and Perspectives' (1985).

8. *Smoking and Health Now*, Royal College of Physicians (1971), p. 59.

9. McKennel and Thomas, *Smoking Habits and Attitudes*.

10. D. D. Reid et al., 'Smoking and other risk factors for coronary heart disease in British civil servants', *Lancet*, vol. 2 (1976), pp. 979–81.

11. J. Nadler et al., in *Lancet*, vol. 1 (1983), pp. 1248–50.

12. W. Baile et al., in *Addictive Behaviour*, vol. 7 (1982), pp. 373–80.

13. J. Deanfield, 'Cigarette smoking and the treatment of angina with propanolol, atenolol and nifedipine', *New England Journal of Medicine*, vol. 310 (1984), pp. 951–4.

14. D. G. Friedman et al., 'Cigarettes, alcohol, coffee and peptic ulcer', *New England Journal of Medicine*, vol. 290 (1974), p. 469.

15. D. J. Smith, 'Absenteeism and "presenteeism" in industry', *Archives of Environmental Health*, vol. 21 (1972), p. 670.

16. W. Willett et al., 'Cigarette smoking, relative weight and menopause', *American Journal of Epidemiology*, vol. 117 (1983) pp. 651–8.

17. C. S. Russel et al. in *British Journal of Preventive Social Medicine*, vol. 2 (1979), p. 231.

18. M. A. H. Russell et al., 'Effect of general practitioners' advice against smoking', *British Medical Journal*, vol. 2 (1979), p. 231.

19. *The Times,* 17 October 1984.
20. C. Brown in *Doctor,* 24 March 1983.
21. A detailed account of these two case histories is given by Peter Taylor in his book *The Smoke Ring.*
22. *Confectionery and Tobacco News,* 6 November 1981.
23. *Health or Smoking,* Royal College of Physicians (1983), p. 98.
24. *Smoking or Health,* Royal College of Physicians (1977), p. 87.
25. *Cancer Research Campaign News,* 13 April 1983.
26. O'Rourke et al., 'Smoking among schoolchildren', *Journal of the Royal College of Physicians,* vol. 33 (1983), pp. 569–72.
27. *Smoking among Secondary Schoolchildren,* HMSO (1983).
28. Survey on the sale of cigarettes to children, Action on Smoking and Health (1975).
29. From a report on a World Health Organization meeting in Colombo, Sri Lanka (18–20 November 1981), to discuss smoking and health issues in developing countries.
30. I. Tager et al. in *New England Journal of Medicine,* vol. 309 (1983), pp. 699–703.
31. M. Kraemer et al. in *American Medical Association Journal,* vol. 249 (1983), pp. 1022–5.
32. *International Herald Tribune,* 6 June 1983.

Index

MORE ABOUT PENGUINS, PELICANS, PEREGRINES AND PUFFINS

For further information about books available from Penguins please write to Dept EP, Penguin Books Ltd, Harmondsworth, Middlesex UB7 0DA.

In the U.S.A.: For a complete list of books available from Penguins in the United States write to Dept DG, Penguin Books, 299 Murray Hill Parkway, East Rutherford, New Jersey 07073.

In Canada: For a complete list of books available from Penguins in Canada write to Penguin Books Canada Limited, 2801 John Street, Markham, Ontario L3R 1B4.

In Australia: For a complete list of books available from Penguins in Australia write to the Marketing Department, Penguin Books Australia Ltd, P.O. Box 257, Ringwood, Victoria 3134.

In New Zealand: For a complete list of books available from Penguins in New Zealand write to the Marketing Department, Penguin Books (N.Z.) Ltd, Private Bag, Takapuna, Auckland 9.

In India: For a complete list of books available from Penguins in India write to Penguin Overseas Ltd, 706 Eros Apartments, 56 Nehru Place, New Delhi 110019.